"I have incorporated Dr. Ries' universal concep
have seen the improvements with my clients. This curriculum helps couples
in all levels of their marriages for both prevention and intervention in the
framework of a critical thinking approach. The book is presented in a
structured, useful, and practical manner and is a great tool for the new or
seasoned therapist looking to work with couples."

– Oudlay Tom, LCSW

"I was first introduced to the Conceptual Template nearly 20 years ago, while
working with challenged youth at a local high school. I was immediately
struck by its direct and positive effect in addressing a wide range of social and
emotional challenges and needs. As I strive to apply the understanding of
these concepts in both my professional and personal life, I continuously gain
a deeper understanding and appreciation of their importance and their
effectiveness in dealing with matters both trivial and profound. Rarely have I
come across a teaching so effective and universally applicable in the resolution of conflict and the promotion of understanding and harmony. I believe
the reader will find the understanding and use of the concepts discussed
within the conceptual template to be most helpful in meeting the inevitable
challenges presented to us by life itself."

– Steven A. Lopes NHD, MA, LMT, Behavioral Health Specialist,
Natural Health Practitioner

"My life was transformed when I learned Dr Ries' Conceptual Template over
30 years ago. I still use his concepts in my daily life with my spouse, children,
friends, students, and even my corporate clients. His concepts and template
help me better interact with the world around me as I practice a more
objectively derived perspective. I have become a more authentic human being
through his work. I find that I can make better decisions, more effectively
manage conflict, better support those close to me, and accept others for who
they are. I highly recommend a deep dive into his work."

– Dr Tim Buividas, partner at The Corporate Learning Institute and
adjunct professor since 1997

Moral Development in Couple Therapy

This innovative text utilizes Kohlberg's stages of moral development, demonstrating how they can be effectively applied to couple and marriage therapy.

Facilitating moral stage development has been found to improve couples' ability to relate to one another, enhancing trust, transparency, communication, and intimacy. Based on empirical research and Kohlberg's classic stages of development, the book showcases the Conceptual Template, a tool for therapists to guide their clients in thinking more objectively about the reality being experienced, their own subjectivity, and how to work together as a couple to mindfully solve problems. With an extensive Instructional Manual as well as a transcript of the author teaching the Conceptual Template process to a therapist, *Moral Development in Couple Therapy* illustrates a highly practical approach to counseling that helps couples achieve a more rational level of moral judgment and reasoning.

Filled with practical case studies and written in an accessible manner, this text is an indispensable resource for couple therapists and other mental health professionals working with couples to resolve conflict.

Steven I. Ries, EdD, is a counselor in private practice on Maui, Hawaii, and was the co-founder and program director of the Human Development Institute in La Grange, Illinois. Previously in his career, he worked as a graduate research assistant under Lawrence Kohlberg at the Center for Moral Education at Harvard University in Cambridge, Massachusetts. Later, Kohlberg became his dissertation committee chairman and Ries graduated with his doctorate from Harvard University in 1981.

Moral Development in Couple Therapy

A New Approach to Kohlberg's Stages

Steven I. Ries

Routledge
Taylor & Francis Group

NEW YORK AND LONDON

First published 2021
by Routledge
52 Vanderbilt Avenue, New York, NY 10017

and by Routledge
2 Park Square, Milton Park, Abingdon, Oxon, OX14 4RN

Routledge is an imprint of the Taylor & Francis Group, an informa business

Library of Congress Cataloging-in-Publication Data
A catalog record for this title has been requested

ISBN: 978-1-138-67810-1 (hbk)
ISBN: 978-1-138-67811-8 (pbk)
ISBN: 978-1-315-55911-7 (ebk)

Typeset in Times New Roman
by Taylor & Francis Books

Contents

Tables

Foreword

Writing this foreword is both an introduction to this book and, in effect, an endorsement for it. Before I rave about the book, let me tell you about my initial conversations with Dr. Steve Ries, the author.

I first met Dr. Ries at the American Psychological Association conference in Honolulu, Hawaii in 2013. My wife, Kathy and I had extended our trip to include a week on the Island of Maui, after the conference when our work and presenting were complete. As it turned out, Steve's home is on Maui, so we agreed to meet up while Kathy and I were there. I met with him first of four times that week in or around his home on the island. Although Steve had spent years thinking about this book, it was during our time together that it emerged from Steve's mind and he spoke about the challenges writing it.

Through the years as a practitioner Steve always wanted to write a book that recognizes and honors his former dissertation committee chairman, the well-known psychologist, Lawrence Kohlberg. I recalled Kohlberg as a brilliant human development scholar, who expanded Jean Piaget's early work in human development. Kohlberg's Stages of Moral Development is a well-known theory in psychology and was best known foremost for explaining moral development in children. Kohlberg was among the first to suggest that this type of development occurs throughout the lifespan and is not limited to childhood.

Either on a picnic table in a beautiful state park or driving around the island, Steve spoke about Kohlberg, moral reasoning, moral development's early formation, cognition, subjectivity and objectivity, and the universal conceptual template that brings it all together. Our conversations made a difference and motivated Steve to return to writing. But what he was actually discussing was how this book would bring Lawrence Kohlberg's theory to new life by focusing on the practical applications with married couples and their moral development.

By the time Kathy and I returned to Honolulu, Steve knew what he needed to do: Write the book. We spoke by phone until he received a contract from this publisher and was assigned an editor. I am delighted to be the first to welcome you to Steve's book.

Steve Ries' *Moral Development in Couple Therapy: A New Approach to Kohlberg's Stages*, is a book, of course, about Lawrence Kohlberg's life work with its inception at the University of Chicago, starting in the mid-1950s and culminating with *The Psychology of Moral Development* Vol. I in 1981 and *The Philosophy of Moral Development* Vol. II in 1984. This book takes Kohlberg's work a step further by applying it to marital or couple relationship and the couple's struggles with moral development. Equally important, Ries notes, is the emergence of an understanding of what is considered fair or just as it applies to working with couples. But it is more than a critique of a well-known theorist. Dr. Ries applies Kohlberg's work to couples in therapy and helps their practitioners in facilitating couples' moral development. Ries's book will bring deserved attention to Kohlberg's life and work and will bring to life his theories through couple therapy.

Within my first year as an assistant professor at Purdue University, in addition to teaching and research I began to see couples at Purdue's Center for Marriage and Family Therapy as a member of the faculty and supervising doctoral students. I was soon working with a reasonable caseload of clients in addition to my clinical supervision. Steve's book would have been an asset to guiding and building clinical skills back then as it is today.

One of my cases during initial practice years was an older couple who had been married for more than 25 years. They also had two grown daughters who were both in college. The older daughter was nearing graduation at the time they worked with me and the other was in the Spring semester of her first year. Neither planned to be living at home after graduation and were out of the picture for our marital therapy sessions during the academic year. We focused on here and now events that helped me evaluate what was happening in their marriage. I saw them for at least seven sessions, every other week until we took a break to see how they adjusted to the treatment. They never returned for any additional counseling, as I had expected.

I thought about this couple from time to time and wondered what else I could have done. After pondering this case for years, I concluded that the key to their marriage surviving the strains they were identifying were reflected in the rudimentary elements they believe in that are contained in their marriage. It was their willingness to face who they are and what they cherish from their marriage both risk and sacrifice. The couple had made peace with their lot in life, I had guessed, and had moved toward a common set of values moving forward.

What we learned from Kohlberg through Dr. Ries's perspectives on couples maturing together is that context is everything, especially in moral decision-making. This goes beyond one's ego to one's oneness/collective/engine/parts of a heart that is connected to their spouse in mutuality. The bond of moral decision-making is the glue that connects and commits couples to each other. My guess is that the couple I worked with so many years ago was dealing with something that had less to do with their love but more to do with their logical or ethical decision-making process.

Dr. Ries's book is a new and exciting approach to healing couples' relationships. He has been able to "pay forward" many lessons and healing strategies, in addition to the tried and true approaches promoted by Kohlberg. The approach builds upon the natural bonds of client couples: Mutual bonds of commitment are the consequences of love, mutual understanding, and respect, along with a dash of patience that comes with time. The mutual commitments of couples also applies to arguments, understandings and truces that emerge during deep conversations together. Ries, being a leader mindful of Kohlberg's genius, effortlessly describes the evidence of morality or moral judgment and reasoning and how it is now viewed as an important cognitive-developmental process. Equally important, Ries explains how the evidence of morality, judgment and reasoning are translated into behavior. Thus, the focus of this book is on the effect of facilitating moral development on intimate partners' interpersonal interaction and behavior.

Ries' Conceptual Template exists for couples to learn how to be conscious and mindful of how they are making a case for the use of knowledge; that the knowledge used is not only to understand and respond appropriately to our life experiences in general. Ries also explains that the Conceptual Template serves as a guide for couples to resolve most conflict between them. In addition, the aim of the Conceptual Template is to facilitate moral development as well as aspects of human development.

My early discussions with Dr. Ries reminded me then and now of the extraordinary legacy of Kohlberg's work. But more profoundly I have been reminded of the power when it is applied to a new context. Couples everywhere have struggled with challenges of the pandemic, illness, death and the changes in their lives to avoid and dread but not each other. In times like these couples have a greater awareness of fragility of life and the power of love in all its stages of development. Clinicians – especially those like me in my early years – will benefit their clients' progress by including moral development in their work with them. Steve Ries' *Moral Development in Couple Therapy: A New Approach to Kohlberg's Stages* reintroduces us all to a kind of wisdom that is timeless and deep in its implications and potential for couples, and that is learning to treating one another with a conscious awareness or mindfulness of what is equitable, fair or just.

Charles R. Figley, Ph.D., Kurzweg Chair in Disaster Mental Health and
Distinguished Professor, Tulane University, New Orleans

Preface

In some sense, it has taken over 25 years to write this book. Kohlberg's research reached its prominence over 50 years ago; nevertheless its impact continues both upon this method of counseling as well as current psychological research in the field of human development. My own empirical research regarding the relationship between self-concept and identity as related to the development of moral reasoning (1979, 1981, 1992, 2006) was inspired and guided by Kohlberg's longitudinal study (1958). The next aspect from which this approach to improving relationships has been constructed is from the philosophical thinking or teachings of great thinkers, such as Socrates, through Plato's writings, Plato himself, and Aristotle. Their contributions were written over 2,000 years ago. It is suggested that these great thinkers' works, including, and, in particular, those of Lawrence Kohlberg, are profoundly important and as relevant today in the field of human development and/or human reasoning as the time period in which they were written, for all people, from all walks of life, cross culturally, across ethnicities, religions, and genders.

This book is written for practitioners, psychologists, and couple therapists, as well as the individual or couple interested in becoming familiar with the construction of the Conceptual Template and its facilitative effect on moral development (Kohlberg, 1958). Detailed information regarding Kohlberg's work, especially the moral stages, will be provided; it has a particular relevance to the clinical application of the Conceptual Template as an approach to counseling couples. This method of counseling, based upon Lawrence Kohlberg's theory of moral development, can facilitate the development of moral reasoning and has been clinically found to parallel improvement of couples' interactions.

The purpose of this book is to introduce an approach to counseling that can facilitate moral development and can thereby result in the positive improvement of human interaction, and specifically, in this case, couples' interactions/relationships. The foundation upon which this book is built is based upon how the mind naturally reasons, interprets, understands or constructs that which is experienced in reality.

Acknowledgments

Charles R. Figley, Ph.D., Kurzweg Chair in Disaster. This book would not exist if it were not for Charles Figley. He more than encouraged me to take on this project. I had wanted to write a book about Kohlberg and moral development and its importance for humanity. I had even spent time thinking about and undertaking this challenge but it seemed as a huge undertaking. Then I serendipitously met Charles at an American Psychological Association Conference in Hawaii. He took an interest in what I had previously written and what I was working on at that time. I was at an impasse and Charles was the catalyst. Charles put what he so insightfully understood about my interest in our short time together and recommended focusing on another important domain in which there was a paucity of clinical approaches to couple and marriage counseling. He offered to work with me, suggested Routledge as a publisher, guided me though the proposal process and even was helpful editing what I had proposed. I often said to him, after he had edited my writing, " Your writing is like magic." Later I "apologized" realizing when being more objective, that what was perceived as "magic," was actually Charles ability, skill and artistic mastery in writing. I acknowledge Charles at length because of having the utmost respect, not only for his writing genius, but also his intuitive insights of my life aim, and perhaps most important, his steadfast concern to be helpful, not only to me but to others in this process. It is then that were Charles to have not existed, or come into my life, this book would not exist. He has never intimated or asked for anything in return. He just gives to help others. When I offered him something for his encouragement and assistance in this project, he said: "Doing this," which he has done for others, is for the reason he gave me: " I sleep well at night." He is a humble man. I too sleep well at night when being so fortunate as to have met such an individual who could read between the lines of our conversations intuiting or rationally comprehending the "trauma" that can lead one to seek justice or love for others because of the value of those who have supported us when having experienced it ourselves. Thank you Charles for standing before me for that which I could not see, and beside me in this challenging and meaningful endeavor.

Elizabeth Graber, editor, who provided guidance with the submitted proposal and contractual agreement as well as in communicating with those involved in such a way that there would be a clear understanding of the aim of this project. Thank you also for spending the time necessary to comprehend the meaning and value of that which was being conveyed while concomitantly maintaining its integrity on the occasion of a more detailed yet concise explanation.

George Zimmar, editor, who early on, in some respects, set the standard of what was expected for this book to be meaningful. His knowledge and experience was sorely missed when he chose to retire. I hope, if he reads this book, that it meets his standard of value.

Clare Ashworth, editor, who kept this process moving at a steady pace while making editorial suggestions that were helpful in creating structure and consistency for the benefit of the reader, for example, summaries at the end of chapters.

Heather Evans, editor, who subtly encouraged me and made editorial suggestions that ultimately, brought this book to fruition. I deeply appreciate all that she has done.

Ellie Duncan, Senior Editorial Assistant to Heather Evans who checked the manuscript to make sure everything necessary was in order before being sent to the copyeditor. Thank you also for your finishing touch and suggestions along with Heather for the most favored choice for a book cover.

Ravinder Dhindsa, copyeditor, who checked for typographical and grammatical accuracy where necessary as well as ensured stylistic consistency.

Kris Siosyte, production editor, who is responsible for ensuring the manuscript being prepared accurately for the typesetter, and who also chose to add italics to specific passages in the transcript for the reader, which clearly brought to the foreground what is essential for understanding and applying the Conceptual Template process. When I first began this book I kept in mind the adage that a journey of a thousand miles begins with the first step, and I would like to especially thank Kris for helping me to complete the last step so that the book is now a book; it is what it is – Reality. Thank you!

My daughter Lisa, an English teacher and published author, for her willingness to edit and revise specific chapters, after "a long day's night" into the wee hours of the next morning. Her knowledge was comforting in not having to be concerned as to her abilities or understanding of what was written, as well as to its meaning and intent. This was particularly important with regard to the "Author's Note" to the reader at the beginning of this book, which was deeply personal. Thank you Lisa for providing me your expertise which I could completely depend upon, having no concerns at all of what you could and did do, which, also reduced some stressful moments in writing this book. I love you!

Thank you, to my son Richard, a licensed clinical psychologist, for his willingness to interpret and assist in the adapted version of Kohlberg's stages. This was, "indeed," at times, a difficult and anxiety provoking undertaking, but at least it is now "extant." Thank you for your Persistence Determination Forthrightness. I love you!

To my youngest daughter Natalie, who will soon also be a licensed clinical psychologist. Thank you for being my personal therapist throughout this endeavor. I love you!

And to my youngest son Nicholas, thank you for maintaining an interest and therefore encouragement in the completion of this project while serving our country in the United State Coast Guard. I love you!

To Dr. Steve Lopes for his thorough reading and understanding of numerous chapters and making suggestions for improving their content to clearly convey the intended meaning. Your friendship as well as your family over the last almost twenty years is especially meaningful to me.

To Ed Rusk, having philosophical conversations with me as well many other dialogues over the last fifty years, and working alongside me in creating our business entity, the Human Development Institute. While what we have done together, as well as discussed over a lifetime are too numerous to even highlight; it cannot be fully comprehended, nor can the extent of our friendship.

However, our collaboration culminating in the Instructional Manual, which ties everything together in such a way that others can learn the Conceptual Template (CT) process, stand alone in its value. Your influence, encouragement, insight, and friendship over the last sixty-five years have value beyond the words expressed here.

Dr. Tim Buividas, once a student of mine, and then early on wanting to work together, which was not affordable, went on to receive his doctorate and opening the Corporate Learning Center. You have in every way possible continued to pursue this goal of working together even at a distance and having separate business entities. You have continued to help and to even mentor me in any way you saw possible to support the ideas of the CT process. No longer a student, you have become a teacher, colleague, and most important, a life-long, loving friend of over forty years.

(Bob) Robert Wiggins Johnson, for his suggestions in writing this book, most notably a comment indelibly embellished in my mind that he taught me, namely, what he learned from one of his teachers, paraphrased, it is: "When you think you have a great sentence, remove it, because it doesn't belong with everything else you wrote." Thank you for your unabated friendship of over sixty-five years

Sue LaFrenz, thank you for your encouragement and support in the value of this process. You have been a good friend, keeping me in touch with reality since we were six years of age.

Bobbie and Brenda Whiteside, thank you for allowing me to use your summer home during the winter months to think and write. It was there on a very cold winter evening that the epiphany of the Conceptual Template occurred.

Thank you to the licensed professional practitioner for revisiting what was initially learned twenty years ago for the purpose of benefiting the reader in better understanding this method of couple therapy. By engaging in this dialogue, you have made more concrete and easier to visualize what could appear for some as somewhat abstract and obtuse. You have, in again going through this process, extended your learning and deeper understanding or knowledge through the meaning of concepts essential to rational and objective thought and specifically with regard to moral reasoning. You have not only gained insight as you expressed, but for other practitioners or individuals to be able to extrapolate this understanding in other domains they may experience. The many hours of your time is appreciated by me and will also be invaluable for those learning to be mindful of this natural or innate process. It can be concluded that essentially what you have taken away from this experience, in your words is:

> It is not just putting your self in another person's shoes and still being subjective. but it is really putting your self in another person's shoes and being objective, looking at objective values and rights… If (couples) learn to just pause and think or reason objectively they would avoid some conflict.

Amanda Marzan was my personal assistant before the onset of this project. When she decided to take on this endeavor, I said what was valued most about her was that she questioned and challenged my reasoning and judgment whenever she had any doubt about the veracity of my thinking. Throughout the course of this project she did more than expected, from being supportive to teaching me things I had not learned in my formal education. For example, when she realized I wrote without having an outline, because I never learned this very important process, she explained to me in order to be helpful, in a quite youthful way that, "First you have to create the skeleton and then put the meat on the bones." While this simplicity could appear somewhat odd to the causal observer of a young person in her twenties saying this to an "educated" individual in his early seventies, it was not. It was her attention to details. It was the willingness to explain or to teach because of her caring of what others might value if aware but do not yet understand or for that matter notice. It is sensitivity and compassion that exemplifies and characterizes who Amanda is. She listens attentively, constructs the meaning of what is said, questions and verifies whether her interpretation is true, and then, with understanding, directly and with as much clarity as she can muster, addresses the issue at hand, for the sake of another. This rational and stoic ability and self-discipline also has at the core of her person a deep sense of empathic awareness as well as a naiveté of the expectation of individuals having equal respect. And, this equality, by extension, wishfully anticipates what ought to be, that is, others to understand and to respond in like kind. Her being rational and objective to a great degree, nevertheless realizes the idealization of her being, and responds, as we all do, in accordance with our self-concept whether in the particular or universal, paralleling our cognition and moral development. In essence, my view of Amanda is that of an enigmatic genius who will, if she has not already, contribute to humanities enlightenment in a most meaningful and significant way by, for one, having helped and guided this book to its fruition. I express this because Amanda's humbleness and to some extent being ego-free, cannot without contradiction realize how others whose eyes doth not rove, with eyes wide open to see, her breath breathes throughout and between the lines that create the meaning of this book. Thank you Amanda!

Thank you to my mother and father for parenting and loving me. In meditation your memory kept me in balance with the rudder of Alfred Sorenson, aka Mr. Nobody, who said, that he "had nothing to say or to teach" when living in silence for forty years in the Himalayas. After reading my dissertation, however, he expressed to me that what is now known as the Conceptual Template "is necessary for people to understand, in order for them to 'innerstand'." An awareness of self and morality, being inextricably intertwined, can result in a mindful and universal understanding or "innerstanding" of all others that equally respects the dignity of each of us, that is justice.

Thank you to my sister Ursula (Uli) for her continued support or encouragement by asking me every time we had a conversation, "What is happening with your book; when will your book be finished?"

To Lawrence Kohlberg to whom this book is dedicated, and would not exist were I to have not had the privilege of his unwavering acceptance, support, guidance and teachings while being my dissertation committee chairman and his friendship until the end of his life. This book is one aspect of how I interpreted what he said to me: "Go out there and do this" when referring to the findings of my dissertation.

Author's Note

This note to the reader is about a young child, who, because of his older sister's experience in school, was excited about the prospect of attending kindergarten. He imagined a day in the near future, either running full speed or, with a little more imagination, riding one of his father's horses to the wooden schoolhouse just down the road; he thought, I can tie the horse to the bike rack. While I know that he also spent much time in the early evening imagining how to build a wooden ladder to climb up to the moon, I do not know what he was imagining, and I do not think he could have imagined that on a warm and sunny day, a seminal event would happen, changing his life, literally, forever. I am aware, however, of what he thought subsequent to this life-altering beating by an older and stronger boy while a younger sister put the finishing touch to this violent act by then kicking this slightly built, and what appeared to be, helpless child, who had understood nothing else in his innocence other than love. That metaphysical perspective was abruptly brought into question. "Why would anyone do such an inexplicable and inequitable act upon another?"

He walked home with some discomfort. He was, for the most part, confused and perplexed, his questions overshadowing what had just happened. His mother welcomed him in her loving manner. He was hurt to some degree both physically and mentally; some might think spiritually. I think not; I know not. Nevertheless, in utter bewilderment, he did not understand the reason that his mother did not say a word to him, other than her usual greeting. Later, when his father returned home from work, having been told of the day's events as always, he also said nothing. What was this child to think?

He thought, "Why did this happen to me?" and "Why do my parents not say anything to me about what happened?" They surely knew. He learned over time, when there were other such occurrences, stemming from or related to this life-changing event, and there were many, that his immigrant parents never said even a word about these similar experiences either. Experience, for whatever reason, if for no other reason, other than reason itself, would be his teacher from that time forward. It was reason that was to address and resolve these evolving questions. "Why do people do the things they do?" "Why do people sometimes harm others, and for what reason?" "What is their reasoning?" And, there remained one last question, the result of the older boy, now a young man, coming to the place where this younger adolescent now worked, to apologize. This led to further and relevant questions. "What caused this change in him?" "What causes change in the way a person thinks?"

These unanswered questions that occupied his mind throughout his youth were not reflective of his parents not teaching him about life. They just did not discuss these types of issues. He later learned that it was because of their horrific experiences and escape from the Holocaust, in what was then Nazi Germany. They did, however, teach him to be respectful of others, particularly to them, and more specifically to his mother and to "girls." That he be respectful of his mother was actually never a concern. It was unnecessary; it was self-evident. Why would he think otherwise of someone who was so sensitive to his needs and wants? She loved him and cared for him with every breath she took, even her last.

After her death, he was sad and angry. After all, it was perceived as a severe injustice in this young man's mind of nineteen years, his mother being "taken" from him. How could He do that?

It would have been preferred by this author that his note to the reader were to have been more light-hearted. Certainly, the perceived injustices to this person – even though for him deeply felt, and as said earlier, were life alter- ing – have but little comparison to those who have suffered or suffer from the magnitude of much greater inequities or injustices that, by chance, a child or person can be born into, or are the result of individuals who have not devel- oped to an adequate level of moral reasoning and know not what they do. For those least fortunate, who do not have freedom, opportunity, or in other ways have been abused or violated, not having their dignity respected, this is acknowledged. That said, to have less severe life-changing experiences by injustices should also not be minimized as to their possible importance to the individual, and are recognized as significant nonetheless. As Dr. Martin Luther King Junior made us aware, with a slight modification, "An injustice anywhere is injustice everywhere," or in his exact words, "An injustice any- where is a threat to justice everywhere." But, this author is neither attempting nor meaning to covey the magnitude of injustice in the world as he may per- ceive it, nor is it the particular reason for this note to the reader. This note is simply a narrative of the journey of a young man who understood, from an early age, the saliency of injustice, or for that matter, justice.

Morality is often misunderstood with respect to its objective meaning and value in the world in which we live. Having an understanding and conscious-awareness of moral judgment/reasoning and its critical beha- vioral effect on human interactions and, in this instance, to the interaction of couples, can bring to light its actual value for all of us.

Fortunately, in spite of the perceived "injustices" that this young man experienced, initially in early childhood, then with the loss of his mother and consequently failing out of the University he was attending during his freshman year, he expressed as a young adult to those close to him that he would, nevertheless, not have wanted to change anything in his life. He also reflected that he did not know whether or even if he would have wanted to change the course of his life if he could, because life seemed to be somehow guiding him. He felt little control in what appeared to him to be a journey and a life worth living, even with, to some extent his perseverating about injustice and justice. The construct of morality seemed to be evolving as a central theme; it occupied his identity, and at times, in his mind, it appeared to be his destiny, even though he did not believe in destiny, per se, or for that matter magical thinking.

Fast forward: he met a witch. Yes, you read correctly; it is a noun and not misspelled, even if, and even though, she never said anything about an ability to cast spells. She was a professor in graduate school for clinical psychology at a university in which he had enrolled. One day after class she said to him, "I am a witch," then clarified, "a *good* witch," perhaps differentiating good from bad because of the concerned look on his face. While he did not believe in witches, witchcraft or witchery, she was bewitching, so to speak.

She then said, "You *must* apply to the doctoral program in Human Development in clinical psychology at the University of Chicago."

He said to her, " I could never get into that school; my grade point average is not high enough."

She responded, "You will be accepted. Apply now, before it is too late!"

He was spellbound, in some sense, certainly dumbfounded, but he immediately applied, and he was accepted.

Shortly thereafter, he was invited along with faculty to an impromptu and unexpected presentation by Lawrence Kohlberg. It was then, at this pivotal moment, that this student realized that all of the questions and the reasoning underlying the knowledge he was seeking since early childhood was a shared experience manifested in the incarnation of a beautiful and loving man explaining his theory of moral development.

Introduction

My Journey with Lawrence Kohlberg

In the 1970s, when I was a graduate student in the Department of Human Development at the University of Chicago, I was invited to attend what appeared to be an impromptu conference in which Lawrence Kohlberg presented a history of his longitudinal research in moral development. Morality had been a particular curiosity to me since early childhood. Prior to Kohlberg's presentation, I had expressed this interest to the Chairman of my Committee, asking to do research specifically regarding the question of whether or not morality and identity or self-concept was interrelated. Hearing Kohlberg's presentation and also having a specific interest in morality, led me to being particularly intrigued by what he had to say. For that reason, shortly thereafter, I contacted him and asked if he would be willing to meet with me. He seemed to have little or no hesitancy and agreed. Our first meeting was remarkable; it was as if my childhood dream were coming true.

Very early in my childhood, during my elementary school years, approximately at the age of eight or nine, I had frequently been intrigued by pictorial advertisements of the Great Books of the Western World produced by Encyclopedia Britannica in collaboration with the University of Chicago. Later in life, after entering college, I noticed two volumes of Plato's writings from this set of classical books on another student's dresser; he allowed me to borrow them. From that time forward, the Great Books became a significant aspect of my education, life, and also my relationship with Lawrence Kohlberg. During our initial conversation, there had been, from my perspective, both an explicable and inexplicable connection, which proved, over time, to be meaningful for both of us. The first connection had to do with my fascination and continuing life-long interest in the Great Books of the Western World. I learned from Kohlberg that first day that the undergraduate liberal arts program at the University of Chicago from which he had graduated was the basis for this Great Books program. The second connection, which Kohlberg and I had, is what I believe to be the effect of this form of liberal arts education. It can encourage a person to be more consciously aware, more mindful, especially about morality.

Whether my perspective of our connection is correct or incorrect, these similar experiences appeared to have created an immediate and somewhat intuitive understanding of one another. And, although our relationship appeared unique and special, my experiences over a decade with other students and colleagues who knew or worked with him, brought to light that, they, too, felt similarly. But for me, my personal experiences with Kohlberg as a trusted friend and mentor, as well as being the Chairman of my doctoral committee, was my childhood dream – of being among supportive and similarly interested individuals – literally coming true.

As our conversation drew to a close that first day, he handed me a many paged book and said that I should read it and come to a seminar the next morning. My impression was that he wanted me to read the book so as to be able to participate at the seminar. I believed, at that time, that it might be a determining factor of whether or not I would be accepted into the Department of Moral Education. After the seminar, it also occurred to me that this experience might also be indicative of what would be expected of a graduate student at this school. This sense of the future was reinforced at the seminar; it seemed apparent that if accepted into the doctoral program, it would minimally require commitment, arduous work, and persistence.

I do not recall the exact number of words, of which I did not know the meaning, let alone the correct spellings, but there were many. Such terms as *ontological, deontological, epistemological, metaphysics,* and *meta-ethics* come to mind. At the time, I had no idea what any of these words meant. These words and others were somewhat intimidating to me. They appeared as if they were commonly used words in the seminar and that it would be expected of me to understand, and also to use them, in the future if accepted into the doctoral program at Harvard. The emotional response to the early morning seminar was apprehension, particularly in respect to succeeding in what appeared to be such a rigorous academic program. Shortly thereafter, I was told, and naively believed, that once one was accepted as a graduate student, "they" will not "flunk you out." What was not said, but was later observed, was that what this really meant was that "they" did not have to "flunk you out;" if a student could or did not do the work necessary, it would be self-apparent, and therefore the person would leave on his own accord.

As difficult and rigorous as the doctoral program at Harvard was, because of my intense interest in morality and cultivating the "unique and special" relationship with Larry (Lawrence Kohlberg, or Dr. Kohlberg, as I knew him, preferred to be addressed as Larry), I was committed to being involved in this program. My childhood curiosity regarding moral reasoning was to understand the reasons that a person or persons could mistreat another. Lawrence Kohlberg (to be formal once again), provided a stepping-stone for this life-long interest or questioning in that he had identified and described cognitive-moral stages of reasoning, which, in my mind, could potentially explain much of moral behavior. His research was, to me, personally, the pinnacle of understanding of the reasoning underlying moral behavior. His research suggested that a significant contributing factor to the nature of human relationships or behavioral interaction is a person's moral judgment, moral reasoning, orientation, or their moral stage(s). These events and that which occurred from that time forward, laid the foundation for this book.

My interest in what I thought to be inextricably tied to our morality, that is, our self-concept or identity, was initially more intuitive conjecture than based upon any substantive objective evidence, until one day, overhearing Larry speaking with colleagues about the phenomenon of moral relativism as being a potential transition from Conventional to Post-conventional moral judgment/reasoning, I saw that a potential connection existed. What was being said that specifically peaked my interest was that some moral relativists in Kohlberg's longitudinal study were at the same time experiencing an identity crisis. I finally had what appeared to be some concrete indication that morality, albeit moral relativism/moral reasoning, and self-concept or identity were, or appeared to be, related. This overheard discussion set the stage for my preliminary research, the purpose of which was to explicate the implications of the psychological phenomenon of moral relativism and its association with self-concept or identity in the process of cognitive-moral development. It was found in this initial study that self-concept, the phenomenon of moral relativism, and stages of moral judgment/reasoning were inextricably intertwined (Ries, 1979, 1981, 1992/2006).

What I also heard that day, which later becomes critically important to what will be presented, were specific philosophical words and concepts. These words seemed to stand out even though they appeared to be casually embedded in the sentences of Kohlberg and his colleagues when portraying the experience of individuals who were morally relativistic, immersed in identity confusion/questioning, and considered to potentially be in transition in their moral development. These words were no different than what Erikson (1968) or any other individual or psychologist with knowledge of identity issues might have used in their sentences when characterizing this phenomenon, or for that matter, perhaps, moral relativism. What was striking, however, was that these specific philosophical words/ideas were seemingly not the major concern to these very erudite individuals. They were used in what appeared to be a more or less conversational way with regard to the subject matter, and were merely necessary in their sentences for the discussion at hand. The casual manner could be attributed to the fact that, in some sense, these specific words actually circumscribed to some extent the experience of individuals in the midst of an identity crisis. Or, that for Kohlberg and his colleagues, it was in fact, a casual and informal conversation while nonetheless important. In a sense, to me, they were discussing the abstract forest of identity crisis or identity confusion as well as moral questioning/confusion, and what I heard, or perceived, were that specific trees, or very concrete ideas, were embedded in this forest. These ideas were truth, knowledge, opinion, belief, objectivity, subjectivity, value, rights, morality and justice. I thought that these very specific ideas/concepts involved in identity questioning were more than descriptive, that they were perhaps essential to the cognitive process of resolving confusion, in general, and, more specifically, identity and moral confusion. And further, I thought that perhaps replicating this process, using these ideas in some form of intervention, could "naturally" facilitate moral development, and in particular, Post-Conventional moral reasoning/judgment.

Mentioning to Larry what was noticed when overhearing the discussion, I suggested that perhaps these specific philosophical ideas/concepts questioned in identity confusion and moral confusion, were in and of themselves essential, or critically important, and needed to be understood by individuals in crisis in order to resolve both their identity and moral concerns. That is, by being able to consciously understand, or conceptualize and then use these ideas in what appeared to me to be a natural occurring process of rational thought, in an integrated way, individuals could make their life experiences more intelligible. And further, thereby, perhaps this could lead to development to Post-Conventional moral reasoning as had occurred with some of his relativistic subjects in their naturally occurring process of cognitive-moral development. This query to Kohlberg led to another concern in the preliminary research (1979), which was to determine if individuals who possessed a qualitative indication that they were in some form of identity crisis were concomitantly also confused with regard to morality, even perhaps specifically being morally relativistic. This research sought to determine if their confusion involved very specific ideas regarding belief, reality, truth, knowledge, subjectivity, objectivity value, morality, and justice as Kohlberg's subjects did. Namely, it was also the purpose to clinically observe and note in this preliminary qualitative study if these individuals specifically and unknowingly, or unwittingly, mentioned or indicated that these specific ideas were prominent in their questioning/confusion. Lastly, if the latter was suggested, then the next logical questions asked were whether or not their identity confusion/relativism was resolved by using these ideas in some conceptually integrated way. And, did this also lead to moral development?

The finding of this aspect of the preliminary research again suggested that these individuals did use the same or similar ideas in their identity questioning and moral confusion, and also expressed them without provocation, that this form of questioning and the resulting resolution led to what they considered to be a milestone in their personal as well as their moral development.

The findings in the preliminary research, then, led to the hypothesis or question of whether or not replicating what appeared to be a potentially naturally occurring cognitive-moral developmental process through some form of intervention, using these same and what appeared to be essential ideas, could facilitate moral development. But first, the most important question which then required answering was: what is this hypothetical naturally occurring conceptual process involving these specific ideas?

One evening, sitting in the proverbial cabin, which a close friend had said I could use during the winter months to think and write, literally snowed in, by maybe five to six feet of snow, snow drifts from the wind blowing off the shoreline of Lake Michigan, I had what seemed to be an epiphany. I thought: these particular philosophical concepts are like the parts of a puzzle. These specific ideas had struck a chord within me in that I remembered that Socrates, who was Plato's teacher, and Plato's writings, or Plato himself, had also addressed these same ideas/concepts. Aristotle, the pupil of Plato, in what appeared to be in a parallel fashion with respect to the importance of words/concepts in relation to reasoning, or to constructing our experiences, admonished the reader about the importance of definition to meaning, and reasoning.

> If one were to say the word has an infinite number of meanings obviously reasoning would be impossible; for not to have one is to have no meaning, and if words have no meaning our reasoning with one another, and indeed with ourselves has been annihilated.
>
> (Aristotle, 1952)

Were these nothing more than coincidental historical events? It seemed that one purpose of these great thinkers' writings was to discuss certain concepts, to assist the reader not only in making life experiences more understandable or intelligible, but also to realize the paramount importance of morality and, in particular, justice. Since these concepts were presented in different writings, and did not appear to have a particular order, the task at hand was to determine if there was some logical and rational order to them and whether the definitions or meaning of these ideas/concepts were interrelated in such a way that they formed an integrated, rational, non-contradictory way of thinking or reasoning. After a period of time of working on defining the meaning of these concepts and how they might be interrelated, and often relying on the mentioned great philosophical thinkers, the "puzzle" came together in what appeared to be an integrated conceptual framework; it formed a rational, logical, non-contradictory framework, and objective way of thinking, or reasoning.

Using the conceptual framework, or Conceptual Template process as a guide in a double blind study, it was found that conceptualizing and integrating these specific philosophical concepts facilitated moral development

(Ries, 1981, 1992/ 2006). In a follow-up study, it was found that the moral development was maintained, and one person, according to Kohlberg, had developed further during this period (personal communication). Shortly thereafter, when I graduated, Larry said to me, "Go out there and do this!"

It did not occur to me when he said this to think of the Conceptual Template process as having potential application for marital, couple or relationship counseling. Marital, couple, or relationship counseling was never addressed in my clinical experiences. It was not taught or part of the curriculum in the schools that I attended, and internships were devoid of individuals seeking marital or couple counseling. My experiences were with individuals who could "clearly" be described, at that time, using diagnostic terms defined in the DSM-III (Diagnostic and Statistical Manual of Mental Disorders of the American Psychiatric Association). When beginning my clinical practice in 1981, however, there were numerous couples, married and not, who were having various types of conflict or difficulties and seeking psychological help. Although I had not heard of marital or couple counseling, and it was not even a part of my vocabulary, and this was not what Larry was implying in saying, "Go out there and do this," with the influx of couples with a multitude of relationship problems, it became evident that it was incumbent upon me to use the educational tools and knowledge I had to assist them.

While the content, in terms of conflict presented either individually or as a couple, certainly varied, some circumstances being more common and frequent than others in occurrence, they nevertheless were invariably a reflection of a common denominator. This common denominator, although presented in different ways or having differing content, was the concern of being treated fairly. It seemed reasonable then, that what was minimally required for encouraging the treating of one another in a more equitable manner, no matter what content, or presenting conflict or dilemma, or method used by a practitioner, it appeared, to me, to be most important to facilitate couples' cognitive and cognitive-moral development. Based upon the earlier research, it was thought that facilitating cognitive-moral development could result in a couple's reasoning more adequately, and, therefore, could result in the individuals treating one another more fairly. Being able to resolve ethical concerns could enhance a couple's relationship in terms of trust. With greater trust, couples could then be more transparent, better able to communicate, better able to understand one another, and, therefore, potentially have greater intimacy. It was further thought that this approach could ultimately result in the recognition of being deeply valued, respected or loved, because being treated in a just manner respects the dignity and worth of one another.

In order to cultivate this conscious awareness, or mindfulness, Socratic questioning and dialogue are used to cause cognitive conflict and to support more adequate structures of reasoning. A more didactic method is also used to supplement the Socratic approach for further clarification when necessary in operationally defining the concepts, which are considered essential to the aim of this process. With rare exception, if any, is this counseling approach found to be awkward or inappropriate. After all, teaching (as I prefer to call this counseling approach), and using a Socratic method, has value in that the practitioner is not telling the client what to do or how to resolve the difficulties being experienced. The client is figuring it out for herself or himself. And, when figured out for oneself, individually or within a relationship, it can be determined that it works; therefore, it proves itself. Further, it does no harm. Learning to think objectively about one's own subjectivity, as well as the natural subjectivity of others, helps us to better understand ourselves. In a relationship, it also enhances understanding of one's significant other, allowing the partner to be better understood, cared about, and respected. All of which are of value in any relationship, any human interaction. Additionally, the value is enhanced because it places the responsibility on the individuals to do the work necessary; the practitioner's responsibility is to assist couples in becoming aware and understanding the conceptual tools of objective reasoning, which then can be developed as any skill is developed; in this case, it is a process or skill of which we are innately endowed. Finally, and importantly, with this particular approach it is not necessary to understand the vicissitudes of the many and various conflicts in order to help the client(s) to develop the skills and conscious-awareness necessary in the resolution of their difficulties. And, in the end, it ultimately respects their human dignity.

Aim of the Book

With all of the above having been said, it is the aim of this book to fill a void by providing the rationale for linking the highly respected field of moral development to the field of counseling, specifically in terms of developing trust and intimacy in couples' relationships. An understanding of Kohlberg's stages of moral judgment/reasoning as a cognitive-moral developmental process will enable loved ones, albeit somewhat subjectively, to determine their own individual levels or stage(s) of development and then to be more able as a couple to set meaningful goals in their relationship.

Common knowledge and experience in relationships suggests that it is important for couples to have trust in each other. Even the most loving couples find themselves wounded emotionally by conflict; while they look to avoid conflict, it is important to know that when conflict does occur, they can trust that together they can resolve difficulty equitably. This book identifies and applies the principles of moral reasoning and development to help couples communicate and resolve differences more effectively. It is not for counselors and their clients who seek to be guided by a set of rigid rules. Rather, it offers the idea that empathy, guided by mindfulness of the reasoning process itself, gives couples greater freedom, understanding and flexibility in their decisions. The *Moral Development in Couple Therapy* is, essentially, a study in fairness, equality, and trust.

The objectives of *Moral Development in Couple Therapy* are:

a   To introduce a new and useful approach to improving couple relationships.

b   To teach individuals how to apply the Conceptual Template to enhance their own development and relationships through objective thinking.

c   To enable couples to create a healthier relationship based upon mutual respect and understanding.

d   To help couples apply essential concepts necessary for both objective as well as rationally consistent or non-contradictory reasoning.

e   To appreciate the concept of the *faculty of reason* and *rational thought* as a natural process that can be improved as a skill and then applied to crisis situations.

f   To appreciate moral reasoning. How we should treat and be treated by others is extremely important for couples to understand.

g   To enable relationships to grow through reasoning in a rational, logical, consistent, and non-contradictory manner and to express comfort, intimacy and love.

h   To teach couples to apply this process of morally focused thinking and being to all aspects of life that require trust and communication.

i   To support individuals in understanding their natural ability to think, communicate and resolve differences fairly.

j   To enable couples to learn to be conscious of these processes so that they can more readily resolve conflict to their mutual satisfaction.

This is a new way of understanding and measuring couples by their stages of moral development. The book addresses the challenges that arise when they are at the same stage of moral development, or when one is above or below the stage of the other. Couples can move to a higher level of moral development and reasoning; becoming more appreciative of their partnership and one another's behaviors, even if there are subjective differences, which might normally cause conflict. By enhancing moral reasoning (cognitive and cognitive-moral development), the couple, as a team, will be more resilient with the resources necessary to thrive (not just survive) traumatic events and lesser challenges.

Building on the theories of human development pioneers (Piaget, 1932, Kohlberg, 1958, Ries, 1979, 1981, 1992/2006), this book is a contribution to, and application of, the study of human development. The following are the basis of this book:

1. The significance of developmental-structural change in reasoning/moral reasoning (not just superficial change) and its impact on the way couples interact.
2. The couple's evolution through stages of moral development expands their abilities and competencies in solving couple-center challenges often ignored in the past, or that resulted in verbal conflict.
3. The Conceptual Template is a conceptually integrated and logically consistent approach to thinking objectively, rationally and clearly. Couples can use it as a strategy for improving communication and resolving differences in a manner that is considered fair to both people.
4. The origin of the thinking of the book is as old as the written word, as long-standing as the study of logic and reason.
5. The basis of this book is the underlying foundation of the reasoning process itself and applies to any situation. This includes times the couple finds itself in the middle of a conflict, disagreement or emergency that requires teamwork.
6. In circumstances in which a strategy or principle has not been specifically learned in a "what-to-do or how-to" book, the Conceptual Template helps couples build their "moral reasoning muscles." Couples will acquire the ability or means to figure out strategies to solve disagreements in a manner that is just. The Conceptual Template, then, goes one step further to enhance the knowledge one has learned from "what to" or "what not to do" sources. It does this by providing a framework for couples to use in order to better understand not only what they have learned, but also how they can construct effective ways to handle unique experiences that they might not have learned, or that they may have learned and found not to be applicable. It short, the template teaches the individual or couple to reason objectively, under any circumstance(s), and to better understand information from other valued resources.
7. *Moral Development in Couple Therapy*, properly applied, should measurably improve thinking skills and an understanding of a step-by-step process for applying the essential ideas of the Conceptual Template. By being conscious of the process in applying the Conceptual Template, couples will better understand subjective experiences in relation to reality. This can be critical to a couple's communication and resolution of differences.
8. This system of reasoning identifies an objective method for solving problems and making responsible decisions and choices that are considered fair by the couple, even if they were to subjectively disagree.

9. This approach facilitates the development of reasoning, in general, and moral reasoning/development in particular. By becoming consciously aware or mindful of this process the mind naturally uses, individuals learn to think more objectively about the reality being experienced, their own subjectivity, and how to work as a couple to consciously resolve conflict.

Chapter 1

The Science Of Morality

The title of this book, *Moral Development in Couple Therapy: A New Approach to Kohlberg's Stages*, while indicating the substance of the information you will learn in this chapter could be easily misunderstood. This is because of what often comes to mind or the common everyday use, meaning, understanding, or connotation of the word moral. In general, when we use the term moral, we are thinking of right and wrong conduct. Such ideas as honesty, loyalty, being kind or nice, doing unto others as you would have them do unto you, or not cheating come to mind, and are examples of what might be considered to be morally virtuous behaviors. If you have a further interest in morality defined in this way and the difficulties it presents in understanding moral judgment/reasoning developmentally, refer to the studies by Hartshorne and May (1928–1930), Kohlberg (1981). The approach here is to look at the scientific evidence of morality (Kohlberg, 1958), not in terms of what is commonly understood subjectively by individuals, groups, a particular religion, or that which a society or a culture deems as moral or as virtuous, but rather to understand morality or moral judgment/reasoning as being a cognitive-developmental process and how this can translate into behavior, (Blasi, 1980, Kohlberg, 1958, 1969, 1984). The focus of this book will specifically be the effect of facilitating moral development on marital and non-marital couples' interpersonal interaction or behavior.

Kohlberg's (1958) longitudinal research on moral development has described individual's progressing through an invariant sequence of qualitatively distinct stages of moral judgment/reasoning. In order to more fully understand what Kohlberg meant by stage, the following characteristics or criteria are among the more important.

Characteristics or Criteria of Stages

1. They are "structured wholes or form organized patterns of thinking." These organized patterns of reasoning are both more "consistent" and "stable" than disequilibrium between stages.

2. They represent a hierarchy of increasing cognitive differentiation and integration. Therefore thinking at a higher stage reintegrates antecedent stages.
3. They form a culturally universal "invariant sequence." Stages cannot be skipped; individuals move to the next stage forward and never backward. Earlier stages, however, can be used.
4. They constitute a hierarchy of perceived "moral adequacy" such that (with the possible exception of disequilibrium between stages) individuals prefer the highest stage they comprehend.
5. Stage assignment is determined by the ability to not only comprehend, but to also be able to construct that reasoning.

Kohlberg defined or circumscribed these stages as "justice reasoning" or "justice orientations." A listing and brief description of these stages and their corresponding levels are summarized in Table 1.1.

The premise of this book is that by facilitating moral development, couples will treat each other in a more just manner, enhancing trust, communication, understanding of one another and consequently improving their relationship. In order to better understand a couple's moral stage or mixture of stages during the counseling process, a broadening of Kohlberg's scholarly and concise rendition depicted in Table 1.1 can be helpful for those with less familiarity of this domain. This more general understanding and shift in perspective can augment a counselor's capability to assist a couple in their ability to improve their relationship. Needless to say, the better one understands moral stage development the more effectively this information can be used in conjunction with the Conceptual Template to enhance a relationship, marital or otherwise. Therefore, to make more substantive what has been described thus far, an elaboration of Kohlberg's descriptions of stages and their development will follow. The purpose will be to assist marriage, couple, family therapists, those in related fields, and others who have an interest that extends beyond the context of this book to more clearly identify the stage or mixture of stages of couples engaged in a counseling process.

Elaboration of Kohlberg's Moral Stage Descriptions and their Development

The following elaborations of Kohlberg's Stages will be described from the least adequate, Level I, Pre-conventional Stages 1 and 2, through Level II, Conventional Stages 3 and 4, to the most highly developed and integrated Level III, Post-conventional Stages 5 and 6.

Table 1.1 Classification of Moral Judgment into Levels and Stages of Development

Levels	Basis of Moral Judgment	Stages of Development
I	Pre-conventional: Cognitive-moral understanding is framed by the interactions between concrete experiential events, and one's own desires and actions, rather than with insight or interest into others experiences.	Stage 1: Compliance to avoid punishment orientation. *Self-centered and self-serving. *Deference under potentially punitive authority. *Avoidance of accepting responsibility for one's actions. Stage 2: Egocentric self-absorbed orientation. *Moral behavior is that which provides personal gain, or that satisfies what the individual wants. *Reciprocity and equality is in mind only as it reflects one's own side of benefits or interests, when involving interactions or exchanges with others.
II	Conventional: Ethical orientation. Reflects awareness of external standards and others' views. Adherence to fulfillment of social-role expectations guides moral judgment in order to receive approval, or maintain one's duty to rules or laws from a pre-existing social system.	Stage 3: Good-person, "good boy or nice girl" orientation. *Emphasis is on being good, or kind by reputation, and on helping or pleasing others, so as to be viewed as a good, nice or kind individual. *Decisions are made that adhere to a somewhat "superficial" interpretation, seen as representative of general norms in a society. *Moral goodness is rooted more in terms of intentions rather than in terms of consequences. *Boundaries are not fully constructed. Stage 4: Order and authority orientation. *The value of boundaries is comprehended. *Moral reasoning reflects understanding obligations from external and authoritative bodies of thought, demonstrating fulfillment of legal, social and religious expectations, which are viewed from this perspective as being the basis of morality, and the basis for morality. *Rigid adherence to duty is seen as optimal behavior to maintain "the given social order."

(Continued)

Table 1.1 (Cont.)

Levels	Basis of Moral Judgment	Stages of Development
III	Post-conventional: Objectivity orientation. Ethical values are oriented to that which can be objectively interpreted as just, and equitable, in relation to the rights of both oneself and others. Rights are understood as that which humans are entitled to by virtue of their existence.	Stage 5: Agreement or contractual orientation. *Appreciation of the potential subjective arbitrariness of moral reasoning and judgment, such as with the rules or laws of a society. *Obligations are seen in the context of shared values with others. *Reasoning stems from a more complete understanding of morality based upon the recognition that objectively based values are more important than subjectively based values in moral reasoning and judgment, and that most values can be set into a meaningful hierarchy. *Objectively derived values constitute rights of humanity. *Individuals are bound by duty to agreements based upon the will and well-being of the majority (utilitarianism). Stage 6: Objective integrity and values orientation. *Reasoning is objective and supersedes law or authority. *The values of equity and equality are regarded in relationship to fairness for the self and all others. *Decisions take into account justice concerns, through a process of objective rationality, generalizability, and justifiability of moral principles across situations. *Reciprocal trustworthiness, and fair-minded regard direct choices with integrity. This integrity is based upon moral principles that entail, and ensure, that no matter what position a person has in a conflict of claims, even the least advantaged, it will be equally fair or just. Further, that even if there is subjective disagreement, rational, objective reasoning and judgment would result in agreement that the resolution or moral principal in upholding the criteria of reversibility and universalizability reifies it being equally just to all involved.

Source: Adapted from Kohlberg (1969)

Pre-conventional Stages

Pre-conventional Stages 1 and 2 are generally childhood stages. As such, this level of moral judgment/reasoning is not common among adolescents or most adults. Adolescents or adults at the Pre-conventional level of Stages 1 and 2 frequently engage in criminal, unlawful, or amoral behavior causing significant conflict with others. Relationships, marital or otherwise are no exception.

Pre-conventional Stage 1 solely entails the individual's perspective, their wants, needs or interests and how they can get what is wanted, needed or of interest to them. Stage 1 reasoning is unable to conceptualize the viewpoint of anyone other than the self. It is a self-centered point of view. That which is considered to be "right" is simply what is wanted. The reasoning for following rules at this stage is based on the fear of getting caught or avoiding punishment in order to get what is desired. That being said, a person using Stage 1 reasoning may break the rules if they believe they can avoid either being caught, punished or any subsequent negative consequences. There is a trouble-avoiding mind-set. Stage 1 moral reasoning is unable to form non-measurable consequences such as emotional or psychological effects on another. This stage can be characterized as concrete egocentricity.

Pre-conventional Stage 2 continues to be self-centered; however, there are two additional developments based on the forming of a rudimentary understanding of another's perspective. Realizing that others might also have their own self-interest or a different perspective there is now the ability to anticipate, to a limited degree, what others think. This limited understanding can be used to manipulate others, again to get what is wanted. There is also the realization that it is possible to get what is wanted through some form of exchange or reciprocity. Reciprocity can be considered a bargaining tool, for example, you do something for me and I'll do something for you, or it can be considered as a justification for vindictive or retaliatory behavior, such as, if someone does something to me then "I will get even" with them. Self-interested behavior, a rudimentary understanding that others can have a different point of view and reciprocity are characteristics of Stage 2 moral judgment/reasoning.

Conventional Stages

Conventional Stages 3 and 4 are adolescent and adult stages. It is during this time that self-concept based upon a Conventional social role identity is being formed (Ries, 1979, 1981, 1992/2006). Conventional Stage 3 moral judgment or reasoning is characterized by caring and conforming to a society's or a group's stereotypical ideas or perceptions of that which is considered acceptable, expected or "right" social role behavior. Conforming to doing what is considered socially "right," "expected, or "acceptable" is motivated by the need to be viewed or perceived as a good person in one's own eyes as well as in the eyes of others and emphasizes not being "selfish." The perception by others toward the self becomes important as we begin forming identities and thinking about what is of value to one's self. An example of social role identities for women is that of the good girl, lady/woman, or wife, and for men is that of the good boy, man, or husband and this becomes the standard for attitude and behavior. Others coming first, pleasing others and self-sacrifice or altruism are paramount in order to fulfill social acceptance, or expectations of doing what is "right," "good," or "nice" behavior. At Stage 3 the reasoning for how we should act and behave is motivated or highly dependent on how we think or feel and are being perceived by our friends, family, group and society. Further, at Stage 3 we begin wanting an identity for ourselves. Stage 3 individuals want to be "somebody" even if they do not yet know what that means, is, or who they want to be. This causes Stage 3 individuals to respond by accepting socially or culturally generalized identities referred to as social role identities. Social role identities are stereotypical because they are based on the ideas or perceptions of behavior of a society, cultural group or rules, not on a particular person's identity. A result of the Stage 3 tendency of naively following rules in order to be accepted and perhaps seeing that different cultures, religions, or other individuals follow rules which are different than theirs, as well as the naivety of allowing others to take advantage or to be manipulated by them, can cause cognitive conflict potentially stimulating and leading to Stage 4 moral judgment and reasoning.

Conventional Stage 4 is initially characterized by learning to formulate personal boundaries in order to protect oneself from naively being taken advantage of by others. This initial integration of valuing setting personal boundaries is the foundation for the further differentiated understanding of the importance of having and following rules or laws for maintaining a social order in a society as a whole. Stage 4's moral reasoning is reliant on rules and laws to create order but cannot formulate the underlying reasoning or ethical principles behind such rules or laws. At Stage 4, rules serve as a means of providing a standard of etiquette or a guideline for what is and is not permissible by a society, a particular religious institution, or any other significant group. It can appear that there is a type of inflexible subjective reasoning specifically with regard to morality, or moral judgment and reasoning. Extenuating circumstances do not alter the basis of a Stage 4 moral judgment because there is little, if any, questioning of rules or laws. Stage 4's moral reasoning does not yet generate or construct independent ideas of moral judgment by using impartial or objective reasoning specifically in terms of morality. Further, Stage 4 moral reasoning does not yet take into account or has not assimilated that rules or laws are functional only in specific situations and therefore can be restrictive in that they might not and often do not work across all similar circumstances. Consequently, Stage 4 moral judgment or reasoning is limited by not having a more differentiated and adequate cognitive-moral understanding of the underlying ethics or reasons for rules or laws that would allow for a more encompassing universal application in adjudicating conflicts of interests

Post-conventional Stages

Post-conventional Stage 5 moral reasoning builds upon Stage 4's concrete understanding of social or societal values, rules or laws. Stage 5's moral reasoning does this by becoming further aware or cognizant of the inadequacy of Stage 4's reasoning which is characteristically often concrete, inflexible or immutable type of moral judgment or reasoning. Unlike Stage 4's concrete understanding of morality, Stage 5 recognizes that there can be an arbitrariness or subjectivity to Stage 4 moral reasoning in that rules or laws can be and often are indiscriminate to a situation or person. At Stage 5, there is the resolution of the inadequacy of this form of specificity by realizing that there are philosophical principles or reasons underlying the concrete and specific reason for a rule or a law. It is at this stage that there is an actual understanding that rights are not merely a concrete conviction but more abstractly an understanding of the reasons underling contracts, agreements, promises, vows, rules or laws. Stage 4 has a black and white perception that following the laws or "rules to the letter" will resolve all issues or conflicts across all situations. Stage 5 adds the ability of seeing further into the reasoning of rules and laws and acting on the principals or "rights" that a law or rule should protect even if that means adapting or adjusting to a new course of action rather than using the rule's original and more general course of action. Stage 5 is able to identify underlying universal human rights and begins prioritizing values and rights into subjective and objective categories, and scaling lower/lesser ranking objective rights and higher ranking/more objective rights into a hierarchy of importance. The cognitive conflict at Stage 5 leading to potentially developing to Stage 6 is recognizing that objective rights can be of equal importance and the questioning of how to resolve these moral dilemmas equitably. Stage 6 moral reasoning begins to have the ability to resolve conflicts involving objective rights that are of equal importance and being more adept at resolving conflicts between rights in a manner that is equitable for all involved independent of personal or subjective consideration.

Post-conventional Stage 6 moral judgment/reasoning is based upon constructing universal principles of justice. A principle is not meant in this context to be a strong conviction as often used "I would not because of the principle of the matter." A principle in Stage 6 moral reasoning is like a rule, but unlike a rule, which works only in a particular situation, a principle is universal and works across all situations. These principles are that which any rational human being, in a circumstance of moral conflict, not knowing what position they could be in would agree is objectively fair or just for everyone in the situation (Moral Musical Chairs, Kohlberg, personal communication). This would still be the case even if they were to personally or subjectively disagree with regard to equally important objective values; the principle is in other words, equally fair or just for all parties involved regardless of their personal position. Stage 6 moral reasoning/judgment respects the rights and dignity of human beings as individual persons in a manner that allows them to be free to choose to live life according to their own free will, without encumbrance so long as it does not infringe upon any other person(s) higher rights, or objectively more important rights. As said, even in a circumstance of two or more individuals having a moral conflict with equally important competing objective values, a principle can be constructed that is fair for all concerned. Based upon this Stage 6 construct, in order for a philosophical principle to be fair or just, requires two criteria to be met, namely, the choice must be both reversible and universalizable. Reversible means that were any person in the same position as another, or any other in a moral dilemma, including the least advantaged, but not knowing which position they could be in, could not, under this "veil of ignorance" (Rawls, 1971), rationally or objectively disagree with the choice made as being just. Universalizability is merely a counter-check of reversibility in that it simply means that even if one subjectively disagrees with the decision they cannot objectively disagree that the choice is fair or just for any human being in that position.

Summary and Conclusion

Understanding Moral Development and the Value of its Facilitation in Couple Counseling

The cognitive or structural-developmental understanding of moral development as described by Kohlberg (1958) and the latter elaboration of these moral stages is the basic foundation for not only realizing the implied underlying importance of facilitating moral development in general, but more specifically to understand the implicit if not explicit value in stimulating moral development in order to improve the quality of the couple relationship, married or not. The differences or similarities in a couple's reasoning due to their moral development is one of the more crucial elements and prevalent causes for both difficulty as well as harmony in relationships such as marriages; facilitating moral development in order to resolve differences can lead to improved couples or marital interaction or for that matter, any human interaction. The less developed a couple's moral judgment/reasoning the less adequate is their ability to resolve difference or moral conflict in a just manner. Conversely, the more developed a couple's moral reasoning/judgment, the potentially more adequate or better their ability to understand, communicate, and treat one another in a just manner and therefore improve or have a healthier more harmonious relationship.

The purpose of elaborating Kohlberg's erudite definitions of moral stages in a more general way was twofold. First, it was to distinguish an objective scientific understanding of moral judgment/reasoning as a cognitive-moral developmental process from subjective conceptualizations of morality as concrete behavioral virtues. Second, for those who are not or are less familiar with this latter moral domain, it was for the purpose of more readily understanding these structural stages. It is suggested that in this manner there is less pressure for the reader to comprehend the levels or stages immediately. A sufficient understanding will naturally occur with these elaborations as well as with the provision of clinical examples that will follow.

To widen this perspective even further then, clinical examples in the form of scenarios will be presented. These vignettes will concretely show how specific stages of moral reasoning can affect couples' interactions or a marital relationship. In essence they will depict what stages can actually "look like" as they present to a counselor in a clinical context.

Chapter 2

The Underlying Psychodynamics and Interactions of Adult Pre-conventional (Stages 1 and/or 2) with Conventional (Stage 3) Moral Reasoning

A Clinical and Behavioral Perspective

The previous chapter described morality as an unfolding process of developing moral constructs, structures or stages (Kohlberg, 1958). This was done to distinguish Kohlberg's explanation of moral judgment/reasoning as a dynamic developmental process from more commonly held static conceptualizations of morality as the embodiment of specific virtues guiding a person's choices and actions. The stages were presented as Kohlberg defined them in his scientific work. An elaboration of these stages was then introduced to provide a more comprehensive depiction. In this chapter, as well as Chapters 3 and 5, the stages are further elaborated upon so as to be more conducive to guiding therapeutic strategies. These three chapters will describe what is observed clinically during counseling couples counseling that is indicative of particular moral stages. In addition, the psychodynamics of couples interaction at different stages specifically with regard to social role identity or self-concept will be introduced when relevant to particular stages. The intent is to even further extend the comprehension of moral development, its effect on couples or marital relationships, and bring to light what the stages actually "look like" when viewed from a more clinical perspective.

This clinical elaboration of Kohlberg's stages will be depicted through the use of narratives or vignettes that are representative of couple's interaction at differing stages, from Pre-conventional to Post-conventional development. These narratives are actual cases compiled with other impressions from clinical experiences. This was done in order to both maintain anonymity of the individuals/couples and to emphasize certain characteristics of Kohlberg's stages by giving more detailed descriptive representations. The clinical examples will be used to illustrate how individuals at different levels and stages of moral reasoning, experience differing types of conflict within a relationship. Clinically it was found that more highly developed stages of moral reasoning could improve a couple's interactions, enhance marital harmony and relationships in general.

Typical Interactions Between Pre-conventional and Conventional Moral Stages

Scenario 1: Typical Moral Stage Interaction between Pre-conventional Stages 1 and 2 and Conventional Stage 3

This narrative describes a married couple in their early forties who have an adolescent daughter.

On a cold winter afternoon, the wife, who had not been feeling well, asked her husband if he would go out to get her some hot soup. It was later that evening, that he returned with cold soup. She addressed this issue during a counseling session. She expressed to her husband that she was upset because he did not come back right away. He knew that she was sick, hungry and unable to easily take care of herself. The wife did not present this issue with anger but rather she appeared rather timid in divulging this information. Although she expressed feelings of hurt to her husband, she did so somewhat timidly and apologetically. Clinically, having a Stage 3 structure of moral reasoning, the wife would not have considered her actions as "being nice" or "her place" within the confines of her Stage 3 social role identity, "the respectful and dutiful, self-sacrificing wife." Often subtle, these observable behavioral characteristics such as being "kind, nice, altruistic and even submissive" are consistent with "the wife's" Conventional Stage 3 social role identity.

The husband presented a mixture of both Stages 1 and 2 moral reasoning. He had knowledge of her being sick, hungry and unable to easily take care of herself, yet he did not call his wife and further did not come back with hot soup until later that evening. His explanation of his actions or inactions appeared defensive. They were simple, and concrete, expecting her to understand his point of view, although unreasonable (Stage 1 and/ or 2). "I wanted to go to my brother's house to work on my car" (Stage 1). When asked, by his wife, why he did not call to let her know his delay, his reasoning was, "You would have asked me to come home" (Stage 1). It appeared during the counseling session that the husband was ignoring or did not understand the reason she was bringing up this issue or the reason for her being upset.

Consistent with Stage 1 moral reasoning, the individual is unable to form non-measurable consequences. At Stage 1, the husband may understand that his wife is hungry, sick and wants hot soup. However at this stage, the individual is unable to put themselves in the shoes of another or to form or understand, other than to a limited and concrete way, the psychological effects outside of oneself. He may understand, "She wants hot soup," but he did not want to come home (Stage 1). During the session, he responded, "Well anyway, you're sick, why would I want to come home?" (Stage 1 and 2). "Well anyway, you're sick." can be suggestive that he is considering what he may get out of staying home in comparison to going to his brother's house. He again restated that he wanted to go to his brother's and appeared to expect her to understand what he wanted or what was important to him (Stages 1 and 2). As he seemed to expect her to understand what he wanted and that he did get her soup are clinically suggestive of Stage 2 reciprocity. Lastly, although I did not observe or hear the husband being vindictive which would typically be indicative or characteristic of Stage 2 thinking in terms of reciprocity, it could be interpreted or suggestive of vindictiveness when he said that the reason he did not promptly come home, was because, "Well you were sick," seeming to imply it was her fault, or placing the blame on her for his decision and action by saying "Why would I want to come home?"

His reasoning and behavior were void of any elements to indicate Stage 3 and/or 4 moral reasoning or the corresponding Conventional social role-identities associated with these stages, such as being "kind, considerate, or responsibility driven" (Ries, 1981, 1992/2006). From a clinical perspective, his behavior would be consistent and having concurrent elements of both Stages 1 and 2 moral reasoning, exhibiting self-absorbed or egocentric reasoning. He emphasized his expectation, both implicitly and explicitly; he projected that she should have understood how it was more important for him to do what he wanted to do (Stages 1 and 2) rather than to come home with the soup still hot. He did not appear to recognize the importance of understanding his wife's needs or to exhibit any apologetic behaviors. All of these observed behaviors would clinically be suggestive of a pattern indicating a mixture of Pre-conventional Stages 1 and 2 moral judgment /reasoning.

Her behavior toward him was typical of Stage 3 moral reasoning, in that she was consistently being very caring and trying to understand his reasoning or point of view. These behavioral expressions clinically suggest the typical naive kindness and "empathy" emanating from Stage 3 moral reasoning. A week or so before our last session the wife had been hospitalized. She said, in session, that her physician had told her the reason s/he was allowing her to go home was because she would recover and be "fine." She appeared to be in denial of the severity of her illness; she appeared moribund to me. It is possible that her physician might not have told her the truth, or that she might have been either in denial or not telling the truth in order to protect her family from knowing that she was dying (Stage 3). Even so, in her somewhat silent suffering, perhaps to protect others, one can see the emotional power of Stage 3 reasoning with regard to the behavioral caring about others at one's own expense, being self-sacrificing or altruistic.

The wife reasoned purely at Stage 3, with no indication of an antecedent structure of Stage 2 moral judgment or the subsequent Stage 4 moral orientation. For example, it would have been indicative of a Stage 4 moral orientation had her reasoning or behavior attempted to set limits to her husband's self-indulgent reasoning and resultant behaviors. It was, at times, difficult and saddening to observe this type of marital interaction. The husband reasoning at the Pre-conventional moral level of Stages 1 and 2 (self-absorbed or unable to form a conscientious perspective), frequently caused conflict in their communication, interactions and relationship. This caring and conflict-avoidance behavior of the wife, characteristic of Stage 3 would not lead to the cognitive conflict minimally necessary for the husband's moral growth. It could be conjectured, that the psychodynamics of the wife's self-sacrificing Stage 3 moral reasoning and the resulting behavioral interactions with the husband, in part, enabled or contributed to the behavioral continuance of the husband at the Pre-conventional level. This caring and conflict-avoidance behavior characteristic of Stage 3 moral reasoning would most likely not lead to cognitive conflict necessary for moral development either in respect to the husband or herself.

A week after our last session, this person, a wife and mother died from cirrhosis. The daughter asked to live with her mother's sister. Perhaps she was projecting her father's reasoning; the father had expressed his feeling of relief of not having responsibility of his daughter when learning she wanted and to go with someone other than with him. He would then be free, he said; "to do whatever he wanted, when he wanted." These types of verbal statements and behaviors again are strongly suggestive of Pre-conventional Stages 1 and 2 moral reasoning.

Scenario 2: Typical Moral Stage Interaction between Pre-conventional Stages 1 and 2 with Conventional Stage 3 Having Remnants of Stage 2 Moral Reasoning

This vignette describes a couple in their early twenties with two children.

In this example of a couple who sought counseling, the man was a mixture of Pre-conventional Stages 1 and 2 and his girlfriend was predominately Conventional Stage 3 with some remnants of Stage 2 moral reasoning. They resided together with their two children. He was a young man in his early twenties, in a gang, who had, previous to my meeting with him, been incarcerated for both assaulting an individual with a golf club for "bird dogging," a fellow gang member, and then subsequently assaulting the arresting police officer. Incarcerated and then released, he was court ordered to receive counseling. He and his girlfriend, also in her early twenties, had frequent arguments during which he could be verbally and sometimes physically abusive. His violent tendency appeared to be exacerbated because he was unable to get employment. It was difficult to get work because of his criminal record.

The goal with all couples is ultimately to facilitate development to Post-conventional Stage 5 and sometimes to Stage 6 moral reasoning. The reason for this is that, the more morally developed the mind/brain, the more adequately a couple can understand, communicate, and treat one another fairly. In this particular instance however, there were two reasons for not expecting development to Post-conventional Stages 5 or 6 moral judgment/ reasoning. First there was a time constraint, as I would be moving to another state. Second this couple was cognitively "concrete operational" as well as developmentally in the earlier stages of cognitive-moral development, namely Stages 1–3. Facilitating their moral reasoning from such early developmental stages so that they could construct Post-conventional Stage 5 or 6 moral reasoning, particularly within this time frame, even if possible, would be unlikely. I had been counseling him for a month and both of them for almost a year when receiving an offer from the State of Hawaii to the Supervising Clinical Psychologist for Baldwin Complex on Maui. In my estimation it would have taken another year of counseling if it were possible to facilitate their development to Post-conventional moral judgment. Stimulating development to Conventional moral reasoning Stages 3 and 4 for both; however, was considered a reasonable goal as well as a possible and worthwhile outcome.

Through clinical/therapeutic observation of the couple, it was determined that the husband was overtly dominant in their relationship. His behavior in session was often demonstrative of controlling, aggressive, sometimes outright mean and/or vindictive (Stage 2) behavior toward his girlfriend. Vindictiveness appeared to occur, in particular, when she would bring up the issue of money. He would react with anger, justifying his reaction by saying she was always complaining and therefore "deserved it." She would respond in a manner that appeared as though she was attempting to appease him (Stage 3) perhaps being apologetic saying she is just trying to help (Stage 3) or trying to be "nice" to him (Stage 3) and saying that she loved him (Stage 3). She would attempt to be understanding of his frustration and be supportive (Stage 3). Her acting angry or using an angry tone with him was never observed in session. She did not appear vindictive (Stage 2) but on occasion her reasoning could be suggestive of Stage 2 reciprocity. For example, she might say things such as "You should not spend so much time at your parents' house when I have to stay home and take care of the kids" (Stage 2 reciprocity).

Within her Stage 3 moral reasoning, she appeared to be attempting to cause him to realize that his Pre-conventional (Stage 1–2) family members were not a "good" influence. This would anger him, and at times he would be oppositional by not coming home, staying with his parents and leaving his girlfriend without their only shared car (Stage 2 retaliation or revenge) by doing so. She would explain to him that not having a car at her disposal in case of an emergency with the children could result in serious consequences. This manner of reasoning appeared to be her way of trying to persuade him to not act out in a retaliatory way. He would, nevertheless, leave her stranded on occasion (Stage 1 or 2). She would sometimes cry or plead with him to not be "so mean" to her (Stage 3) but rather to be "nice" (Stage 3). There was no indication that she acted differently at home; he complained about her crying and being a "baby, and having to toughen up." Sometimes he would not tell her where he was going so she would not know where he was. It appeared that he did this purposely just because he wanted to (Stage 1) or in order to upset her by being vindictive. He appeared to do this following her complaining about his (Stages 1 and 2) inconsiderate behavior.

Initially, or at the onset of counseling, it appeared as though he was not listening or caring about the Conceptual Template process. Rather he seemed to just be going through the motions to appease the legal system by attempting to get a letter from me for attending counseling. In his way of thinking this would indicate he had fulfilled the court order. Although he was challenging, and at times incorrigible, he slowly and painstakingly was learning the Conceptual Template process. It was around this time that there was also evidence that this young man was seriously attempting on a daily basis to get employment. He often expressed disappointment, that it was unfair, that just because he had a criminal record no one would hire him. He became more willing to learn the Conceptual Template. This was encouraging and after approximately nine months of counseling his moral development was suggestive of Stage 3 moral reasoning. For example, he would apologize to his girlfriend when he reacted with anger and he exhibited less anger over time. He had still been unsuccessful in getting a job, but his girlfriend would express that when returning home, he would comment, "he hoped, she would understand that he was trying" (Stage 3).

He also expressed on more than one occasion at about this time in the Conceptual Template process that he would not give up, that he wanted to be a responsible and good person (Stage 3) with the corresponding social role identity. He would say that he knew he had a responsibility to his children, and to her, which clinically would be considered a Stage 3 response or perhaps even the beginnings of Stage 4 moral reasoning with a corresponding social role identity of provider or breadwinner. Rejected as well as dejected, he continued attempting to convince this one particular business owner to hire him. He told the employer that he had learned from his mistakes and really needed to be responsible in order to support his girlfriend and children. He said that, he promised the employer he would follow the rules of the company (Stage 4). He had also pleaded and told the employer he would never let him down; he got the job.

After a month of work, he bought his girlfriend an engagement ring; shortly thereafter they were married. He purchased a used car, for her. He said that his car was not in as good of a condition as the car he had purchased for his wife but that he could fix his car if it broke down (Stage 3). He often had problems with his car but it appeared he made it to work every day, on time, without incident (Stage 4). He was presenting himself quite differently than he had first presented; according to his wife, he was kind and caring toward her, during as well as outside of our sessions (Stage 3). In addition, early on in counseling he had frequently missed appointments giving various excuses such as, "I forgot" or "I was looking for a job," "My car broke down" or "What good is learning this stuff doing for me anyway?" (Stage 2). Now he no longer made excuses. He showed up at every appointment on time (Stage 3 and 4). He stopped associating with his gang, saying that he "wanted to do the right thing" (Stage 3), and he "wanted to be 'somebody'" (Stage 3 with corresponding social role identity). He talked about his family: one brother hiding, having escaped from jail, his other brother on parole, and his father a career criminal and abusive to his mother. "I don't want to be like them; I want to be a good person" (Stage 3). He appeared to be changing into a "new person" or developing a new social role identity. He no longer fit into the social role identity of a "gangster" and appeared to be adopting or developing into the role of a "good and law abiding person" (Stages 3 and 4).

Several weeks before moving out of state, our sessions had to come to an end earlier than preferred, but we had time to work through important issues. When I told them they succeeded, he started to sob. This was unexpected and surprising; he was a "tough guy," literally and figuratively. He said he would "miss me" implying that he would like to have continued counseling. Upon reflection, much of this was expressive of Stage 3 reasoning and the emotion often associated with this stage. He was in the process of choosing to make important and more mature changes in his life. He was predominantly Stage 3 with some minimal Stage 4 reasoning at our last session almost a year later. This assessment was supported by the observation that he was being more responsible toward his wife and children and that he was somewhat "obsessed" about following the rules (Stage 4) at the business at which he was employed. This was critically important at this particular type of company because of the nature of the work. Any indiscretion could lead to immediate dismissal and perhaps criminal prosecution. Lastly, he stopped going to his family's home except on rare occasions. Giving the reason for this change that, they were all a "bad" influence and did not abide by the law (Stage 4). His wife, at the end of our sessions, was a mixture of both Stages 3 and 4. This couple was not conflict free, but there was apparent improvement in more open communication and understanding, with no obvious evidence of his earlier Stage 2 vindictiveness in moral judgment/reasoning or behavior. It is noteworthy, that retaliatory or revengeful behavior, although more indicative of Pre-conventional reasoning, is not uncommon for persons who are Conventional in their moral reasoning, particularly when emotionally upset, frustrated, or angry. Lastly, there had not been any further mention of him being abusive verbally or physically. This also appeared to be supported in the way he treated his wife during later sessions.

Elaboration of Stages and Underlying Psychodynamics of Both Scenarios 1 and 2

Scenarios 1 and 2 were presented to be representative of couple's interactions when one spouse is Pre-conventional and the other is predominantly Conventional Stage 3 in their moral judgment/reasoning. As characterized in these scenarios, the husbands at Pre-conventional Stages 1 and 2 are individuals whose cognitive-moral development operates solely in a manner concerned with their own wants or self-interests, and have a predominantly self-centered perspective. At this level, their cognitive-moral development suggests simplified priorities and awareness. Pre-conventional moral reasoning can precipitate conflicts in couples or any relationship as its awareness may be described simply as the self and other than the self. Awareness of anything, or anyone, other than the self, is reduced to something or someone to be managed or avoided in order to obtain what the self wants, and to avoid that which is disliked. Adult individuals at Pre-conventional Stages 1 and 2 want to do whatever they want to do, and to avoid that which could impede them from that which they want. For these individuals at the Pre-conventional level, they interpret punishment as merely a hindrance from that which they want to do and therefore dislikeable and something to avoid.

As implied in these two scenarios, adult individual's at the Pre-conventional stages are not capable or do not have the cognitive competence of putting themselves "in the shoes" of others, such as their spouse, or to empathize the emotional or psychological effects, significance or impact of their egocentric behavior on their partner. They do, however, have the ability to concretely identify specific types of emotional responses. They have the experience and sophistication such that they can then use this concrete identification or information to use to their own advantage. For example in Scenario 1 the husband is concretely aware of the emotional response that would occur if he told his wife he was going to his brother's house to work on a car rather than bringing home the soup still hot; she would be upset and want him to come home. Avoiding calling his wife so that he can avoid coming home and go to his brother's house is a clinically observable egocentric behavior typical of Stage 1, and even Stage 2. Stages 1 and 2 are self-centered mindsets, and while Stage 2 may begin to comprehend motives or emotions of other's, this information is primarily constructed as knowledge of what is to be managed to obtain what the self wants or at Stage 1 what is to be avoided to escape the consequences of what the self dislikes.

In Scenario 2 the husband exhibits another important construct of Pre-conventional behavior, which is, reciprocation. The husband gives the reason behind the assault of another person as being, "He was 'bird dogging' my friend" which was another gang member. And, we can again see the consistency of this construct of Stage 2 moral judgment when he had later also assaulted the arresting police officer with the justification that the officer was trying to arrest him. In his Pre-conventional thinking, he had done nothing wrong. In other words he felt justified, because in his egocentric reasoning, the "bird-dog" was deserving of his "lickens" (Colloq.) as was the police officer attempting to arrest him.

Similarly, in Scenario 2, the husband would at times not come home after visiting his parents. He said that the reason he did this was because he was angry at his wife's complaining of his spending time with them. He was simply, in his words, "getting back" as his wife. This behavior can be interpreted as reciprocity taking the form of vindictiveness or being revengeful. In this instance, his revengeful behavior could also be interpreted as manipulative ultimately for the purpose of intimidation. The behavior can also be viewed as emanating from the ability to concretely identify the potential emotional effect and response of his wife, namely, a catalyst or a provocation for his Stage 3 spouse to acquiesce to her Preconventional Stage1 husband's wants.

It is suggested that it is the clinically observable egocentric trouble-avoiding mind-set, reciprocity and frequently vengeful reasoning and behavior of Preconventional reasoning exhibited by both husbands in each of the scenarios that appeared to be the primary cause for significant conflict in their relationships. It is noteworthy for the practitioner that vengeful or vindictive behavior has been emphasized in these vignettes because it is typical, or frequently the result of Pre-conventional judgment in adulthood, particularly when impeded from what is wanted, which is also characteristic of this level, particularly Stage 2 moral reasoning. While violent behaviors in this regard can also occur, there are, as suggested in these scenarios, the non-violent although not always non-aggressive behaviors also consistent with Pre-conventional reasoning regarding reciprocity which are commonly observed at these stages. Behavior consistent with Pre-conventional reasoning is also inclusive of when the individual exhibits "niceness" or offers favors for something they value of equal or greater status in return. The favor is presented with the appearance of an act of kindness or of being caring when in reality it is a subtle form of manipulation for the purpose of some form of anticipated reciprocation.

Relationships of couples such as described in Scenarios 1 and 2, where one partner is Pre-conventional and the other is predominantly Conventional Stage 3 in their moral reasoning, although fraught with conflict, can continue and sometimes does "work" to some degree, but in a dysfunctional way. The reason for this, although somewhat counter-intuitive is both because of the characteristic Stage 3 person's moral reasoning as well as the underlying psychodynamics of one's social role identity. In each of these scenarios, the Stage 3 moral reasoning of the wives is buttressed by the social role identity of being a "dutiful good wife." In the vignettes, as often seen clinically, the Stage 3 social role identity is characteristically altruistic or self-sacrificing. It is kind or nice to a fault. It is giving, helpful, understanding, empathetic, and often appeasing both verbally and behaviorally. With these underlying psychodynamics, it is more under-standable how some of these marriages occur in the first place and con-tinue to "work" even if riddled with conflict. The social role identity entailing self-sacrifice, always wanting to be helpful and caring can be an "ideal" spouse for a Pre-conventional, predominantly self-serving person. Conversely, for some individuals, in my experience many, who are Stage 3 in their moral reasoning with the corresponding supporting social role identity of nurturing, giving, and in so being, wanting to help by changing a person who is Pre-conventional, can initially appear to be optimal to them as well. In short, the characteristics of Stage 3 moral reasoning or a mind still without "borders," or not yet Stage 4 moral judgment, can both allow for and support these dysfunctional relationships.

Summary and Conclusion: Behavioral Interactions and Psychodynamics of Pre-conventional and Conventional Couples

Two scenarios describe the stages of a Pre-conventional spouse with Con-ventional partner in moral judgment/reasoning typical of what is observed clinically both verbally and behaviorally. The interactive nature of these particular stages, there underlying psychodynamics as well as how differ-ences in moral development frequently appears in a clinical setting was also addressed. These scenarios, contrasting a less adequate with a more morally adequately developed spouse had the purpose to widen the coun-selors understanding of moral development and stage, that is, in general. The purpose of presenting these scenarios, contrasting a less developed and more developed spouse, with regard to moral development, was to broaden the counselor's clinical understanding of the said stages in cou-ples. And, more specifically, it was the intent to extend the counselor per-spective and ability to not only identify the stage(s) of moral development of those with whom s/he is counseling but to further understand the effects of less adequate stage development on the nature of couples interaction. More specifically, the intent in presenting these scenarios was to broaden the counselor's perspective and ability to not only identify the stage(s) of moral development of those with whom s/he is counseling, but to further understand the effects of less adequate stage development on the nature of couples interactions.

These first two scenarios, as will those that follow, are for the purpose of making even more apparent that which might initially appear obtuse with regard to understanding moral stages and their development. The next chapter will identify typical clinically observable characteristics of couples that are both at the Conventional level of moral reasoning and the nature of their interactions.

Chapter 3

Typical Interactions Of Couples Conventional In Moral Judgment/ Reasoning

The preceding chapter contrasted the moral development of two couples viewed from a clinical perspective. Two individuals, both Pre-conventional (Stages 1 and 2), and their spouses who were Conventional (Stage 3) were summarized through the use of scenarios demonstrating the nature of their behavioral interactions typical of these stages. This chapter similarly focuses on typical interactions of a couple; however, in this instance, both individuals are Conventional Stages 3 and/or 4 in their moral judgment/reasoning. It will be shown and implied, that conflicts in Conventional moral relationships substantively differ from what is commonly observed when one of the individual's in the relationship is Pre-conventional, as indicated in the previous chapter. In addition, since understanding social-role identity's relation to moral development can also explain some of the underlying reasoning affecting individuals' or couples' interactions, it will also be discussed when relevant.

The aim of this chapter then is to again further clarify and broaden the understanding of what Conventional moral stages can look like, and/or the nature of behavioral interaction as observed and interpreted in a clinical setting. This broader clinical framework can be of value in that it can provide further substantive information to assess the underpinnings of couples' interactions, which can then be used by the mental health practitioner for furthering couples' development. This information can also assist couples when this book is suggested reading as part of the counseling process. And, for those individuals who are not engaged in counseling, but nevertheless have found interest in this book, it can provide additional awareness for improving their ability to more objectively understand and communicate with one another in a more intimate manner.

Typical Behavioral Interactions at Conventional Moral Stages 3 and 4

Scenario 3: Both in their Early Twenties, a Couple after Having Been Married a Little Over Three Years Came in for Counseling

They were both predominately Conventional Stage 3 with some adjacent Conventional Stage 4 in their moral judgment/reasoning. They viewed and called themselves "good Christians" (social-role identity). This suggested Stage 3 moral judgment/reasoning with a corresponding social-role identity of being "a good person, husband or wife" (Ries, 1981, 1992/2006). Both the husband and wife consistently presented as very "nice" people and pleasant in manner; their behavior was considerate and caring about each other's feelings (Stage 3). They showed no animosity throughout the several months of counseling, or any form of resentment toward one another (Stage 3). There was no evidence of verbal or behavioral vindictiveness or abuse (Stage 2) or the slightest evidence of hostility directed toward one another even though they had wanted to be divorced for approximately two years (Stage 3). The behavioral interaction described thus far is not meant to imply that this couple never had conflict under different circumstances, but rather that being nice, kind, or trying to please one another is typical of Stage 3 moral reasoning with its corresponding social-role identity (Ries, 1981, 1992/2006).

This couple literally had a moral dilemma, and did not know what to do about it; their dilemma was that they were no longer romantically in love and therefore wanted to divorce. Initially, divorce had not been considered because both they and their parents strictly upheld and adhered to the tenets of Catholicism (Stage 4). Divorce was therefore untenable for them. Further, they indicated not wanting to hurt their parent's feelings or to disappoint them (Stage 3). They believed that their parents would not have accepted their "disobedience" to the orthodoxy of their religion (Stage 4). Additionally, being a " good Catholic" (Stage 3) was part of their social-role identity. They believed that they should remain married, and by the time they initiated counseling it was too late for an annulment within the framework of the Catholic religion (Stage 4).

Both individuals' expressed their deep love of God, Catholicism, the Church (Stages 3 and 4), and their parents (Stage 3) as well as to each other (Stage 3) although in a non-romantic way. They were young adults, naive, nice, caring, wanting-to-please and self-sacrificing, all of which exemplified Stage 3 moral reasoning concomitantly juxtaposed with abiding the laws of Catholicism (Stage 4). With these structures of reasoning in place, and having to somehow be reconciled with their not wanting to be married because they simply did not love each other in "that way" anymore, was a very perplexing and morally conflict-ridden problem for both of them to resolve.

They perceived and had also described themselves as "nice" people (a Stage 3 social-role identity or self-concept) and not wanting to hurt anyone's feelings (Stage 3). This was consistent with their identity or self-concept of being "good Catholics" or good people in non-denominational social-role terms. Choosing divorce would not only bring their social-role identities and corresponding Stage 3 moral reasoning/judgment into question or conflict, but further it would also contradict the laws of their religious teachings or beliefs (Stage 4). After several months of counseling, they decided that they had no other rational, objective alternative choice other than to dissolve their marriage, otherwise they would continue to be unhappy in their lives. They explained to their parents their reasoning, and were "forgiven" by them (Stage 3).

The cognitive conflict of their moral dilemma alone might have been a stimulus for furthering their moral development. In this instance, however, the conflict was resolved in a caring Stage 3 manner. Stage 3 moral reasoning/judgment is consistent with those aspects of their parents' reasoning as well as those aspects of Catholicism that can also be of a Conventional Stage 3 moral orientation, such as, forgiveness. From this perspective, all involved were able to maintain their self-concept, or social-role identity of being "good Christians." Further they could consider themselves to be moral, kind, and caring, people (Stage 3) while following an aspect of Catholicism that for them meant that they were not outright disobeying the laws of the Church (Stage 4). They were able to resolve their ipso facto moral dilemma or conflict in a way that could offer them contentment under these difficult circumstances. Following the rules of their religious denomination (Stage 4), "Christianity," coupled with the Stage 3 orientation of being nice, caring, or understanding, as well as the corresponding social-role identity of being a "good Christian," all contributed to this couple's civility toward one another and having conciliatory sessions. When these Stages 3 and/or 4 behaviors consistently occur, it suggests that an individual or a couple is at the Conventional level. The above scenario conveys what moral conventional orientation "looks like" from a clinical perspective.

In that facilitating Post-conventional moral judgment and reasoning can, and usually is a goal of the Conceptual Template approach, a preferred or more adequate outcome for this couple's future from this perspective would have been that they resolved their moral dilemma by having developed to Post-conventional Stage 5 moral judgment/reasoning. However, learning to be conceptually conscious of objective reasoning occurs in the first half of this counseling process or what heretofore will be referred to as the Conceptual Template model. Once this process of objective reasoning is understood, it is then applied, in the second half of the Conceptual Template, to moral judgment/reasoning for the purpose of both facilitating moral development (Ries, 1981, 1992/2006) and thereby improving couples' interaction. This couple had resolved their moral dilemma during the first half of the Conceptual

Template paradigm and felt there was no further reason for marital counseling. Counseling ended shortly past the midpoint of the Conceptual Template, that is, prior to its application to moral development. Nevertheless, the first half of the Conceptual Template was beneficial in that, it was instrumental to these individuals in facilitating objectivity in their rational thought, and specifically with regard to their awareness of subjectivity as applied to the concern or issue of whether or not dissolving their marriage could be morally possible within the context of their life circumstances.

The couple also came to their own conclusion and resolution using predominately Conventional Stage 3 and 4 moral judgment, that divorce was the only objective way for them to resolve their moral dilemma operating on the premise that each acknowledged their individual "right to happiness" beyond fulfilling their parents' expectations or perhaps even those of the Catholic church. At Stage 5, the elements of the scenario could have been similarly resolved, but the reasoning would have differed. They would have made the decision with the underlying structure of moral reasoning that what is "right" so to speak for them, is their actual individual right in reality for freedom and happiness (Stage 5). The decision would have been independent of their parents' approval (Stage 3) and again Catholicism (Stage 4). It would be unlike or dissimilar to Stage 3 moral reasoning wherein there would be reasoning indicative of dependence on their parents' or religion's approval as a justification. In other words, the underlying moral structure would recognize theirs as well as others inalienable right to their own existence or life, which is inclusive of their right to freedom of choice and the pursuit of happiness.

We can also glean, to some degree, from this clinical example, the characteristic stability of Stage 4, both in moral reasoning and its subsequent effect on behavior. Stage 4 moral reasoning/judgment clearly circumscribes and sets limits on behavior. It has greater adequacy than Stage 3 in its comprehension of the value of constructing rules for the purpose of order and agreement. It is this ability and recognition of the greater adequacy of setting limits on behavior that can lead to Stage 4 moral reasoning. In other words, it is the resolution to the conflict inherent in Stage 3 moral reasoning. As mentioned earlier, a person having the underlying structure of a Stage 3 moral orientation will act in a manner that they think will please others. Their reasoning is less oriented to what is "in their best interest," but rather more so in the interest of others. The reasoning is based on what is "nice" or again, likable or pleasing to others. This may lead to situations that can be disadvantageous and/or unfulfilling. Stage 3's self-sacrificing and people pleasing reasoning, can be described as naive or simplistic in moral judgment/reasoning because it is undifferentiated in having not yet recognized the capability and full value of setting limitations on their own or others' interactive behaviors.

The Stage 4 rule-oriented person is capable of constructing boundaries or limits of behavior. Family, peer groups, society, culture, ethnicity, religious groups all provide their own influences on an individual and a couple's morality or ethics. The confines of socially acceptable and expected behavior in social relationships such as how a father is expected to "bring home the bacon," so to speak, or a mother expected to put supper on the table at a particular time are examples of the type of basis for which we might begin to construct a social-role identity. Stage 4 acknowledges and understands the direct relationship of setting boundaries or limits of behavior not only for social order but also to avoid situations that can be disadvantageous and/or unfulfilling for one's personal preferences and/or well-being or self-image. From a clinical perspective, it is noteworthy that this seemingly "matter of fact" aspect of a Stage 4 rule-orientation, can have the appearance of a more rigid reasoning and behavior, or "being set in one's ways." Social-role identities corresponding to a Conventional Stage 3 moral orientation seem somewhat less stable in the clinical sense, in that the person behaviorally attempts to adjust to others in order to both avoid conflict and to be liked by being nice, caring, and understanding.

While all of the above clinical analyses are to a greater or lesser degree generalizations, they can nevertheless be helpful in identifying the predominant moral stage(s) of reasoning. And, since behavior has been contextually linked to moral development in this clinical analysis, it cannot be emphasized enough that Kohlberg's identification of stages and their development, were first and foremost descriptions, not prescriptions, that is, in the sense of to what individual's ought to adhere. Kohlberg's stage description were however, implicitly prescriptive, in that each stage within the invariant sequence of development has greater adequacy in terms of moral reasoning (Kohlberg, 1984, p. 293) as well as behaviorally (Blasi, 1980).

I would like to end this chapter by pointing out that Kohlberg's stages having been described by him as descriptive, rather than prescriptive, or being used as judgments of the individual as a person. The first time I heard Kohlberg state this idea was at a conference at a medical school. Kohlberg was asked if his Moral Judgment Interview and scoring of the stage(s) could be used in screening potential medical school applicants. Kohlberg replied, that just because an individual is or is not at the highest stage(s) of moral development does not mean that this person would or would not be an excellent physician. While I thought I understood the meaning of his statement, I only realized the full extent of what Kohlberg meant later while teaching a child psychology course at a community college. Having brought my oldest daughter to class, as an example of a child who was developmentally Stage 1 and/or 2 in moral reasoning (moral stage development had been previously discussed at length in earlier classes), a student asked me, "What do you think of a Stage 1 and /or 2 person?" I was somewhat stunned and taken aback for a moment, at what

I emotionally perceived to be a potential insensitivity to my daughter's feelings, but also to not having words to respond. I realized that I had apparently not thoroughly thought through what Kohlberg had said about moral stages being descriptive. But, I collected my wits, seriously thought about the student's poignant question, and finally realized with what appeared to be all eyes in the classroom on me, including my daughter's, and then said with conviction, "Well my daughter is stage 1 or 2, and I love her." Having said this, and so as to not misunderstand Kohlberg's intention with regard to his stages being descriptive, it is also important to be aware in couple counseling that while a normative Pre-conventional child does not differ structurally from a Pre-conventional adult who is Stages 1 and/or 2 in their moral reasoning, a Pre-conventional adult's behavior as compared to a child, is critically important in comparison, particularly when working with adult couples and the nature of their behavioral interaction. This is because of the potential degree of the consequences or effects of a Pre-conventional adult's behavior on others as compared to a child as illustrated in Chapter 2.

The purpose of this chapter was to highlight and contrast the differences in behavioral interactions of couples in which one is Pre-conventional Stages 1 and/or 2 in their moral judgment and the other Conventional Stage 3 in their moral reasoning, (as described in the previous chapter) with a couple in which both were Conventional in their moral reasoning (Stage 3 and Stage 4). By comparing and contrasting Chapter 2's couple, one of which was Pre-conventional and the other Conventional in their moral reasoning, this chapter also illustrated that facilitating moral stage development of couples to predominantly Conventional Stages 3 and 4 in moral judgment/reasoning can potentially improve overall interaction.

Lastly, transitioning from Conventional to Post-conventional moral reasoning has been historically an infrequent event, but is ultimately the intent of this counseling approach. According to Kohlberg (personal communication), only 15% of individuals naturally develop to Post-conventional moral reasoning; 12% develop to Stage 5 and 3% to Stage 6 moral judgment/reasoning. From our discussions as well as my own preliminary research (1979), which, in part, involved autobiographical as well as biographical material of individuals who appeared highly developed in their moral reasoning, it was also indicated that Post-conventional moral reasoning was historically rare and further was preceded by identity and moral confusion during transition (1979). While this transition to Post-conventional moral reasoning appeared rare, it was also suggested by the preliminary research findings that identity and moral confusion associated with moral development if resolved could potentially result in Post-conventional moral judgment/ reasoning. Later research in a double blind study (1981, 1992/2006) supported this idea that resolving existential confusion and issues regarding identity and morality frequently (40% of morally conventional subjects) resulted in Post-conventional Stage 5 moral reasoning. In our conversations Kohlberg and I had often discussed what appeared to be an increase in moral questioning/confusion as well as existential questioning/confusion. The 1960s through the 80s were a historical period of time that generated and supported both existential questioning/confusion as well as many young people's rebelliousness toward conventional morality and the questioning of their own identity and morality. These latter events seemed to be associated with the occurrence of the injustices of the Vietnam War. Since this appeared to be a phenomenon that in our history ushered in both questioning and confusion of moral and identity concerns for many, and for some, development to Post-conventional moral judgment/reasoning, Chapter 4 will briefly describe this time period. This next chapter will serve as a foundation for the scenarios in Chapters 5, which will depict couples' development to Post-conventional moral reasoning.

Summary and Conclusion: Couples' Behavioral Interaction at Conventional Stages and 3 and 4

This chapter focused on the use of a modified clinical analysis in order to give a more detailed behavioral description of the Conventional orientations of Stages 3 and 4. Based upon clinical observation, it appears that Pre-conventional moral stages have a propensity to actually create conflict to a greater extent than behavioral interactions at the Conventional level. This clinical analysis will hopefully provide the mental health professional further insight as to the importance of understanding the developmental succession of stages in order to use this information to facilitate the progression to higher stages of moral development, with the potential result of improving marital harmony.

The intent was to distinguish behavioral interactions of couples having the underlying structure of Conventional Stage 3 and/or 4 moral reasoning, as compared to having the underpinnings of the antecedent Pre-conventional stages.

Chapter 4

Historical Events of the 1960s and 1970s Affecting Moral Development

There have been numerous events dating from the 1960s to the present that specifically affected moral development. Notably during this time period, the questioning of conventional society in general, in particular, the questioning/confusion of both one's conventional identity or social role identity as well as conventional morality stand out. This questioning of societal norms was, to some extent, socially and politically interpreted by conventional society as rebellion. It nevertheless resulted, for one, in the strengthening of the women's modern-day movement toward greater gender and social equality. And, it has, to this time in history, further strengthened the naturally occurring human potential for moral development toward a Post-conventional orientation.

Women, who had traditionally manifested the stereotypical social role identity of being the nurturer and caregiver during their relationship as a couple, began questioning and frequently continue to question to the present their social role expectations. The "Me Too Movement" of today is one result of this cultural phenomenon that exemplifies the extent of this idea. In particular, the idea of women being submissive, subservient, or being quiet with respect to what some think is an aspect or an expectation of their social role is being responded to by encouraging speaking out assertively against injustice, *in this instance, sexual harassment.* These social role identities of being the "nice 'girl'," "good wife" or, for that matter, the "good husband" significantly corresponds with stabilization in Conventional moral reasoning/judgment Stages 3 and 4 (Ries, 1981, 1992/2006). Women have historically tended to be predominantly Stage 3; however, since the 1960s, a phenomenon has occurred in which many women began to progress either to or through Conventional Stage 4 moral reasoning toward an intuitive sense or a comprehension of Post-conventional Stage 5 moral reasoning. This development appeared to also coincide with women more clearly sensing or realizing their self-identity and/or self-worth, dignity and rights (Ries, 1981, 1992/2006). Many women became more assertive in expressing what they perceived as just. They advocated for a more egalitarian relationship as a couple, in their marriages, and other relationships, as well as in their professional life.

Nevertheless, women early on during this potentially transitional time period often continued to be predominantly Stage 3 in their moral judgment/reasoning with the corresponding behaviors, as they were just beginning to assimilate Stage 4 moral judgment/reasoning. Cognitive-development and cognitive-moral development are a relatively slow process of assimilation and accommodation that universally proceeds ontologically in an invariant sequence of stages. We all go through these stages a step at a time; we cannot skip a stage, although reasoning can be used from any stage we already understand. For example, a person who is predominantly conventional in their moral reasoning could potentially revert to a Pre-conventional form of reasoning and behavior, under stressful conditions. Each stage is logically built upon the previous one and this process takes time. Therefore, as women have progressed in their moral development, many did not have the sufficient time necessary to fully assimilate and accommodate, or to integrate the next moral stage. Many women were not completely out of Stage 3, while having already begun to construct Stage 4 and concomitantly questioning and confused with regard to conventional or traditional ways of thinking, including their traditional social role identity or self-concept. Women's unfolding development was being stimulated in part by the Women's Movement during the 1960s continuing to the present, by being in the workforce, and experiencing the cognitive conflict all of this can entail. The workplace is in general a Stage 4 social environment, in which an individual is immersed in a societal perspective vs. a Stage 3 perspective, which is that of a participant or individual being a member of a group. Stage 3 is partial in perspective; it takes into account the personal individual's perspectives, whether with regard to one's self or that of others. Stage 4 is more impartial in that it can consider the general, group or societal perspective. There is greater variety, opportunity and frequency of occurrences that can create cognitive and cognitive-moral conflict in the work environment. This can lead to constructing boundaries or rules and thereby facilitate the development of Stage 4 moral reasoning. The construction of boundaries or rules creates a foundation by which to build a perspective of how they believe they should behave, and how they believe others should behave toward them. Again the present day "Me Too Movement" is an example of the effect of the strengthening of the women's movement.

Women then, were to some extent assimilating, understanding, integrating and developing to Stage 4 moral judgment/reasoning. And, some women, as said, even began to grasp a sense of or construct Post-conventional Stage 5 moral judgment/reasoning. Post-conventional Stage 5 moral judgment and reasoning, again, was also found to significantly correspond to a self-concept which was no longer identifying with a conventional social role identity, but rather a more universal conceptual understanding of self as "being a person" (Ries, 1981, 1992/2006).

On the other hand, the "good" husband of today appears to have most often developed and stabilized at a Conventional level of moral judgment/

reasoning, particularly at Stage 4, perhaps with some minimal or marginal Stage 3 remaining. Being predominantly Stage 4 in moral judgment/ reasoning corresponds with the social role identity of provider (Ries, 1981, 1992/2006). The "man of the house," typically the husband, has traditionally been in charge of the nuclear family. He was the bread-winner, and this had been the socially expected family construct. The social construct of "The man of the house" traditionally entails making the rules and creating order in the family. It is conventionally con-sidered the responsibility of the dominant figure to be both the provider and protector, even if passive in behavior.

Before the 1960s, men appear to have had not only a more clearly defined social role identity but also a more clearly defined structural and stabilized form of Stage 4 moral judgment/reasoning. The catalyst for this was their historically earlier and greater exposure to the "outside work world." The work world functions for the most part in Conventional Stage 4 terms, "laws and order." The idea of men being "the nurturer and care-giver" in the family was not a social construct at that time. To some extent, the husbands' Stage 4 moral reasoning and social role identity today is like that of their predecessors. They continue to see themselves as the provider and protector of the family and are most frequently Conven-tional Stage 4 in their moral judgment/reasoning. Unlike the husbands before the 1960s, however, it appears as though, husbands since the 1960s have a less clearly or "rigidly" adhered to, or circumscribed Stage 4 moral orientation, having more remnants of Stage 3 moral reasoning existing than their predecessors. The occurrence of this phenomenon of a lingering Stage 3 morality and self-concept is perhaps because men are now expec-ted to shift in their social role identity to be the caregiver or nurturer (Stage 3). This has been occurring more often as women have increasingly gone further in their education, have more commonly entered the business or work world, and perhaps even become the sole provider, for one, because they can sometimes earn more income then their spouse.

In the 1950s then, men had a more rigidly defined social role identity as well as a more clearly defined Stage 4 Conventional form of moral judg-ment/reasoning. The 1960s and all that has evolved from this period has appeared to have ushered in a "new" way of thinking. Husbands today, although remaining stabilized at Stage 4, clinically appear to have more elements of Stage 3 than their predecessors, with a paralleling social role identity. They can be more flexible and responsive with regard to their own willingness for development when seeking assistance through counseling than men who in a previous generation were both conventionally and/or structurally stabilized, and therefore perhaps, characteristically more "rigid" in their orientation. Lastly, husbands of today also clinically appear more accepting, willing or open to their spouse's continuing development, per-sonally and professionally.

The effects of the1960s events on couples or marriage is perhaps most profound in how it has affected human behavior in general, and relationships in particular. The results of this historical phenomenon, of questioning social constructs, including civil rights, of social role identity, self-concept and conventional morality are what is clinically observed both during this time period and subsequently when counseling couples. It is most evident in the greater frequency of moral subjectivity and its extreme form of moral relativism, which impacts not only an individual's moral judgment/reasoning but also couples' behavioral interaction.

The Historical Events Of The 1960s and 1970s Affecting Conventional Moral Stages 3 and 4 Reasoning

The effects of the 1960s and 70s can be further illustrated as before through the use of scenarios. This is clinically important to understand both because it is so prevalent and it can be an opportunity for the practitioner to augment or encourage this process already in progress in constructing the most adequate or developed stages of moral development, namely, Post-conventional Stages 5 and 6. Comprehending and utilizing Post-conventional moral reasoning can have a dramatic effect in that it can ultimately increase the mind's cognitive adequacy in resolving all types of conflict and the ability to resolve complex conflicts of interests more equitably. This process is supported during counseling by the use of the Conceptual Template.

Scenario 4: Typical Characteristics for the Potential Transitioning from Conventional to Post-conventional Moral Reasoning of a Couple in their Mid-forties Having Both a Late Adolescent Daughter and Son

When I initially met this couple, the husband, who was from an island in Southeast Asia, was identified as a mixture of Conventional Stages 3 and 4 in his moral judgment/reasoning. Although living in America, he was steeped in the cultural milieu and expectations of the country in which he had been raised. The ideology from that culture, and expectations in terms of social role behavior for a woman/wife had not had the historical changes as manifested in Western culture's Women's Movement of the 1960s. It continues, although somewhat attenuated, to be the norm for a woman of his birth country to be Stage 3 in moral reasoning associated with and supported by her traditional social role identity as the "good, nice and self-sacrificing woman/wife." In his culture it is considered unusual, aberrant, and somewhat frowned upon behavior if a woman does not maintain the social role identity of the "good wife," the nurturer or caregiver associated with Stage 3 moral judgment/reasoning. Women of his native background provided support to their family but were rarely heads of the household and were also more characteristically appearing submissive as well as dependent or reliant. This was in stark contrast to his American wife's moral judgment/reasoning who was a working business owner and independent thinker. Even though she too was a mixture of Conventional Stages 3 and 4, unlike her husband, she had adopted some of the characteristic ideas typical of transitioning to Post-conventional Stage 5 moral judgment/reasoning. Her Stage 5 ideas included her rights and independent thinking as an individual autonomous person. This was in part a result of identifying with her father who encouraged autonomy and the Women's Movement of the1960s. Although she was a mixture of both Stages 3 and 4 moral reasoning, neither was predominant. Her moral reasoning fluctuated depending upon the issue. There were also indications that she was questioning the subjectivity of both Stages 3 and 4 forms of reasoning. She appeared to be experiencing identity questioning and possibly an identity crisis/confusion as to her "identity" or her "social role identity." Identity questioning is among the particular types of self-introspection that can be a catalyst for a potential transition to Post-conventional (Stage 5) moral judgment and reasoning (Ries, 1979, 1981, 1992/2006). This possible transition that she appeared to be experiencing, with its associated behaviors, was a major source of conflict in their marriage.

She was becoming more independent, enjoyed spending time with her female friends and co-workers, sometimes going away for a weekend camping with them, or going out after work. To her husband, she appeared somewhat irresponsible. At times during our sessions, she would verbally appear, in content although not structurally, to be using Pre-conventional Stage 2 moral judgments such as saying "I should be able to do whatever I want." Another reason it was hypothesized that she was perhaps in transition to Post-conventional Stage 5 moral judgment/reasoning was because of the Stage 2 content interspersed within her questioning of her Conventional Stage 3 and 4 underlying moral structure. Indicative of a transition to Post-conventional moral judgment/reasoning is that the content of what is said can sound as if it is Pre-conventional Stage 2 (Kohlberg, personal communication). It is, however, too sophisticated and philosophically oriented to actually be Pre-conventional (Kohlberg, personal communication). Her expression of her ideas and justification of her behavior was quite philosophical, again raising the question of whether she was or was not, actually in transition to Post-conventional moral judgment/reasoning.

She had already asserted herself in society, having opened her own, now a successful business, and had for most of her life, according to her, been "independent" because she "identified" with her father and his encouragement for her to be autonomous. She discussed her lifelong rebelliousness, emanating from being independent, as encouraged and supported by her father. Also, even though she was too young to directly experience the 1960s, she was nevertheless indirectly influenced by this "time period," the music, the idea of "Make love not war" and to doing what one wanted to do, to be "free." Her idea of freedom did not have the constructs or structure of a Post-conventional Stage 5 understanding, such as rights. To her, she had the "right" to do whatever she wanted, when she wanted, even with her understanding of Stage 4 moral reasoning. This was also one of the reasons she questioned her Stage 4 thinking; it contradicted her modus operandi. She said that she felt constrained by her marriage and felt aspects of her marriage were contradictory to the idea of being "free." She was philosophical about her thinking, expressing what could be interpreted in content to be hedonistic, and self-centered ideas (Stages 1 and 2). Although what she often said appeared in content to be of a Pre-conventional genre, it was the underlying reasoning and her awareness of her own and others' subjectivity in which she seemed to be keenly interested that suggested she was potentially in the early "stages" of assimilating Post-conventional moral reasoning.

Her awareness of subjectivity also suggested that it might be an opportune time to intervene with the use of the Conceptual Template. Awareness of one's own and others subjectivity is also characteristic and necessary to transitions to Post-conventional thinking. She just did not have, as yet, the conceptual tools necessary to be able to construct Stage 5 moral judgment/reasoning; she was confused about her marriage and her social role or identity as a wife. She just wanted to be "free" as she appeared to have, from my clinical perspective, interpreted her younger impressions of what was occurring historically during that time.

Her husband had at first appeared somewhat resistant to learning the Conceptual Template. He was, in a manner of speaking, trying to "hold on" to his idea of a traditional marriage of many years. He had thought it was a good marriage. He stated that he was a responsible husband and provider (Stages 3 and 4) and that he never went outside of what he considered to be the sanctity of their marriage (Stage 4). His Stage 3 caring, being a nice giving person (Stage 3) even altruistic at times (Stage 3), his love and respect for his wife, the results of this way of thinking and his flexible attitude softened the edges of his Stage 4 moral judgment/reasoning. It was possible because of all of these factors to create a somewhat philosophical dialogue between husband and wife. This type of interaction had not occurred earlier in their marriage but both were willing to engage in this kind of dialogue using the Conceptual Template as a guide. The result was ultimately that both developed to Post-conventional Stage 5 moral reasoning although it was more pronounced in the wife's moral reasoning. She made this transition within a somewhat shorter period of time than her husband, again suggesting, post-hoc, that she was indeed approaching a potential transition as earlier hypothesized. Although it took him more time because he was not in transition but rather was stabilized at Stage 4 with residual Stage 3 remaining in his moral judgment and as part of his identity, that is, of being a nice person, as said, he too eventually developed. They have now described themselves to be very happily married. She told me at the beginning of counseling she "could not stand" the way her husband "looked," and other descriptive phrases of not wanting to be physically near him. She said, "I just want to get away from him." At our last session, she stated that she "loved her husband more today than she ever had because they communicate better, have a more intimate understanding of one another, and ultimately have a greater respect and love for each other as individual persons." She continues to go camping with her female friends and co-workers, or just goes out to have fun. Her husband, understanding Stage 5 moral reasoning/judgment regarding rights said that he no longer had an issue with his former concern or expectation of her maintaining a social role which he had been accustomed to in the culture in which he had lived most of his life.

By extrapolating this couple's interactions, which are specific to their experience, through the use of an imaginary scenario, it can be illuminated even further what may happen and has frequently happened somewhat typically in other Conventional Stage 3 and 4 couples' relationships.

Imaginary Scenario

The scenario, although imaginary is again a compilation of what I have most commonly observed in couples counseling; being less specific can be more easily generalized. The scenario will feature a couple where the man is predominantly Stage 4 with some remnants of Stage 3 and the woman is predominantly Stage 3 moving to Stage 4 and sometimes intuitively sensing Stage 5. In my experience, this has been a frequent occurrence since the 1960s, 70s and early 80s where couples have some measure of conflict because of differing stages as well as the potential historical effects of this time period. In my clinical experience, there is a more frequent occurrence of women developing past Stage 4: This scenario begins with a couple in which the wife is moving from Stage 3 to 4 moral reasoning and the possible conflict between her and her husband that can occur because of her development.

As a woman develops past Stage 3, she begins to assert herself, even if initially in a somewhat timid way. She might ask her husband permission to do things before actually making her own decision. She might say, "I have to ask my husband first" when deciding on something that could be considered trivial. The husband can and often does become upset or distressed at the changes that can begin occurring in the household. He can try to assert himself in a dominant manner over her perhaps using words such as, "I am head of this family" or "This is my house." He may try to reason in such a way as putting himself in a more powerful position because he is the man, provider and more physically domineering. At

Stage 3, an individual is somewhat characteristically altruistic; a woman is generally a social role oriented wife. She cooks, cleans, takes care of the children and most often thinks of others before herself because a social role oriented wife is stereotypically sweet, caring and altruistic. At Stage 4, the convention has been that the husband takes care of his family financially, is the head of the family even if passive in nature, and often has the final say or "word" on decisions of what is "best for everyone." It can be disorienting for a husband when a wife starts to have an opinion for herself with regard to finances, house or family rules and "what is best for everyone." A husband can, and frequently is, disrupted in his idea of his home and his family when a wife begins transitioning from Stage 3 to 4 or even more so to Stage 5. For example, the wife wants to start her own business. Using Stage 3 reasoning a husband may fear for her. He might be concerned that others will take advantage because of her lack of experience with people that do so. He also may experience a type of insecurity as the head of the household and can react at times by being unsupportive or gruff, easy to anger and disengaged with both her achievements and hardships. "It was your decision; you deal with the consequences (Stage 4)." Love can soften the edge at times of this struggle where the husband is supportive and caring (Stage 3) of his wife and she is empathetic over his personal insecurities of his social role identity as husband or provider and "man of the house" (Stage 3).

The growing independence of the wife and her achievements as a provider or co-provider of the family continues with new challenges. The wife may want to go out with her co-workers or friends after work and let off some steam. She may avoid going out with her friends for fear of upsetting her husband (Stage 3). She may go out with her friends but only once in a while with the permission of her husband in situations that are conventionally considered acceptable such as work conventions (Stages 3 and 4). At Stage 5 the wife asks her husband if she can go out with her friends once in a while, but is able to understand that she has a right to enjoy herself as long as it is not at the expense or rights of her family.

In this imaginary scenario going out one evening with her friends does not appear to be an infringement upon the rights of her family or her husband; however, the husband is now alone with the kids. It is possible that this is the first time he is responsible for planning a meal for the children. The kids are tussling and arguing while he prepares the meal, being challenging and a handful as children sometimes are. He may scold them and tell them to set the table both to contain them in an acceptable alternative as well as to maintain order (Stage 4). They finally sit at the meal table when one announces that they do not "eat" this type of food. The girl is allergic to mushrooms and the boy doesn't want to eat his vegetables. It can be disheartening to a father who just realizes that he does not know all the intricacies of the children as his wife does. He tells his daughter he will make her something else that she is not allergic to and orders the son to eat his vegetables or go straight to bed (Stage 4).

The wife comes home from her night out with her friends. The husband is surly from a difficult and eventful night. An argument ensues. The husband wants her to stay home as before. He doesn't want to have to stay home with the kids while she goes out. The wife reacts saying that he sometimes goes out fishing with his buddies on the weekend and she should be able to go out too. He can feel like the family life he has known is changing and it is not what he has come to expect from their former traditional lifestyle. She used to stay home with the kids, taking care of their home and he would be the one to work and provide for the family. The "normal" order of things is changing and it is uncomfortable for him. Meanwhile she can feel the need for independence, respect as a person, and flexibility and support from her family, especially her husband. Both can feel that this is not how it should be, that is, the fighting and the possibility that they cannot resolve it.

Summary and Conclusion

This chapter very briefly described the historical period of the 1960s and 70s in order to suggest or indicate its effect on human development, particularly with regard to potentially leading toward Post-conventional moral reasoning. The chapter also described both an actual, although modified case scenario, and an imaginary one. The couples in the two examples were at the Conventional level experiencing what appeared to be a dynamic disequilibrium. It was suggested that this disequilibrium was a result of the questioning of both Conventional morality brought on by one or both spouses potentially transitioning to Post-conventional morality and their corresponding conventional social role identities. It was further suggested that this form of a spontaneous and dynamic disequilibrium of previously stabilized stages was a result of the events occurring during the 1960s and 1970s. It was also implied that this phenomenon and the use of the Conceptual Template could potentially lead, in large measure, to the transitioning from Conventional to Post-conventional moral reasoning. This is critically important to understand because, for one, the effects of the 1960s and 70s are still common and therefore continues to be an opportunity to augment or encourage this process when already in progress, toward the more developed stages of moral development, Post-conventional Stages 5 and 6. Most importantly, comprehending and utilizing Post-conventional moral reasoning can have a dramatic effect on a couple's ability to increase the mind's adequacy at resolving all types of conflict including but not limited to individual temperance during disagreements and the ability to resolve complex conflicts of interests more equitably. This process was supported, as mentioned, during counseling by the use of the Conceptual Template.

In both Scenario 4 and the imaginary scenario of this chapter it was implied that there is both the potential for moral development, to create, and even increase conflict in couples' interaction when this dynamic cognitive-moral disequilibrium is occurring, such as by effects of the events occurring during the 1960s and 70s and the later aftermath. It was suggested that an increase in conflict can lead to difficulties other than those of fairness in couples' relationships, particularly if one reaches Post-conventional moral reasoning and the other does not. However, it is also possible, that since cognitive conflict is a necessary condition for moral development to occur, even if not necessarily a sufficient condition, that moral conflict can also be an opportunity for growth or further development. In Scenario 4, in which the Conceptual Template was the modus operandi of the therapeutic process, the couple had the opportunity to use this objective way of reasoning to enhance their relationship where both parties could experience fully communicating and appreciating one another as individuals. Scenario 4 illustrates a couple that was experiencing conflict. They were able to develop and enhance not just their communication and attraction but to also reconnect emotionally as well, saving their marriage. Implementing the Conceptual Template, then, as suggested in the last scenario, can stimulate moral development and lead to a favorable outcome. The scenario in the following chapter will similarly describe another couple having learned the Conceptual Template also to have a favorable outcome in their relationship.

Chapter 5

Post–Conventional Moral Development Facilitated through the Implementation of the Conceptual Template

This chapter, like the preceding one, suggests that recognizing and questioning the subjectivity of Conventional morality or social constructs as occurring during the 1960s and 70s, and consequently questioning one's own identity and morality, could potentially have been a natural catalyst for facilitating moral development, specifically, to a Post-conventional orientation. The latter chapter as well as this one, each depict a couple, in which one individual in the marital relationship indicated to have been affected by the events of the1960s and 70s, and at the time of counseling clinically appeared to also be potentially transitioning to Post-conventional moral reasoning; the other individual in each of these relationships remained stabilized in Conventional moral judgment/reasoning. This difference in moral judgment and its behavioral manifestations caused significant conflict in the relationships, resulting in couple counseling. The Conceptual Template, which conceptually represents what, appears to occur naturally in cognitive and cognitive-moral development (Ries, 1979, 1981,1992/2006) was used during the counseling process with beneficial outcomes, which will be described in what follows.

In order to further illuminate the potential effects of the Conceptual Template process in regard to couple counseling, this chapter goes one step further. Rather than providing clinical interpretations or analyses, the couple in this chapter is asked three questions specifically about how the Conceptual Template process affected them. These questions were asked after a period of time after counseling ended. It was requested that the responses be done independent of their spouse and to be responded to in writing. Therefore, when these questions are addressed in this chapter, they are verbatim.

This scenario involves a married couple. The wife was formulating Post-conventional Stage 5 and her husband was Conventional Stage 4 in his moral reasoning at the onset of counseling. Both were quite reflective thinkers and independent individuals. A few years after counseling ended they gave permission for their story to form a scenario as well as provide personal information in response to three specific questions in a follow-up interview subsequent to the intervention of the Conceptual Template paradigm. The following will depict the intricacies of their relationship both during and after counseling. The purpose will be to delineate challenges that can ensue when one spouse has reasoning that is Post-conventional and the other spouse is Conventional (Stages 3 and 4) in their moral judgment. It will also indicate that when using the Conceptual Template as a tool in facilitating moral development to Post-conventional moral reasoning, it can potentially lead to improved communication, understanding, as well as a more equitable relationship.

Scenario 5

At our first meeting he was fifty-two, and she was forty-five years of age. They had three children ranging in age from ten to sixteen years. He was a successful businessman. She was also successful in the field of education as a teacher. The wife had naturally developed from Conventional Stage 4 to having some Post-conventional Stage 5 moral reasoning prior to marriage counseling while her husband was stabilized in Conventional Stage 4 moral judgment/reasoning. The difference in their moral developmental stage(s) was an evident and significant source of conflict.

In this latter context, it is noteworthy that it is important for the counselor who understands moral development as a process, to remember to explain, and to emphasize early on to their clients that all human beings go through, although some further than others, an invariant sequence of stages of both cognitive and cognitive-moral development. Therefore the client, when learning about moral development, can be reminded, particularly if judging their partner harshly as being less adequately developed, that we all go through these stages as structurally described in Chapter 1. And, that some stages, such as Post-conventional (Stages 5 and 6) can take a lifetime to understand or to construct or might not to occur at all. The practitioner might give an example to their clients to help them understand the value of understanding the stages as being descriptive of what we all can experience during our lifetime. I use the example of one of my own children, as discussed in Chapter 3.

The problem presented by this couple was the contrast in relation to their expectation of the social role of a spouse. Both of these individuals had a conflict regarding an expectation not being met or being imposed on them by the other. Her idea of what she wanted and expected was so important to her in marriage, that it was preemptively and literally expressed in their marriage vows. It was a poetic excerpt from Kahlil Gibran's book, *The Prophet*, when he speaks of marriage. It's written (p. 16):

> And stand together, yet not too near together:
> For the pillars of the temple stand apart,

And the oak tree and the cypress grow not in each other's
shadow.

She felt, after years of marriage, that what she had valued was being
eroded. She said that her Stage 5 Post-conventional moral reasoning was
to some degree supplanted by ideas associated with the expected Conventional social role identity of what a wife should be and what she should
conventionally value in her marriage.

She was to be, in a few words, the dutiful wife. She worked part-time
with her husband, and was also a teacher. She was taking care of the
children, reading and doing homework with them, preparing meals, as
well as tucking them into bed. This was her expected social role as a
mother.

Although not in the Conventional social role identity of a husband, he
was also at times helpful, for example sometimes cooking dinner, helping
the children with homework or tucking them into bed. He was an intelligent man who enjoyed reading about personal development. When talking
with him, it appeared that he valued his wife's independence and appreciated her intelligence. He asked her to work with him to help in a new
business venture, mentioned earlier. He viewed himself as the provider,
even though, she also worked full time in addition to her motherly role,
was involved in community work and helped in his business.

Both had a lot on their plates. She was at times exhausted after working, feeding the children, putting the children to bed and other responsi-
bilities before she could rest. Her husband often wanted to be sexually
intimate at inopportune times for her. It was this expectation pushing her
endurance and tolerance that appeared, so to speak, to be the straw that
broke the camel's back. It appeared to her to not be a choice of yes or no,
but what a good, nurturing self-sacrificing wife should do, that is, a rem-
nant of Stage 3 moral reasoning and its associated identity. (We all can use
earlier stages of moral reasoning as earlier mentioned, particularly under
stressful conditions). Thus she experienced cognitive and cognitive-moral
conflict with her identification of this social role expectation of the conventional and dutiful wife and found it to be unjust. In her use of Stage 5
moral reasoning, her vows were a contract of being more or less independent and having freedom of choice. Further, she understood in her Stage 5
reasoning that she had the right to make her own choices limited only by
the priority of a higher right.

Her husband although loving, caring and appreciative of his wife, often
felt frustrated by her occasional avoidance of his sexual advances. It was
difficult for him to comprehend that she was often tired. He too worked
tirelessly having two businesses. They both loved each and got along well,
having other values that were congruent. His internal conflict appeared
clinically to have a more direct relation with the desire to be desired by the

woman he loved than with sexual intimacy. Another possibility of the husband's internal conflict with the pursuit of his wife's affection could be the perception of what rights and autonomous will are, versus wants, and socially expected behaviors or duties. And, without doubt one of the underlying psychodynamics to both his sexual desire and frustration, as he expressed, was that she was "so physically attractive" to him.

She attempted to break away from the social role expectation of sexual intimacy that should not be a wife's duty but rather a physical and emotional expression of love and caring in their relationship. Her husband, at that time, did not fully understand that his wife might not always wish for his physical attention, even after an exhausting day of work or taking care of the family. He "always" felt desirous/amorous for his wife, as they both loved each other deeply. Often enough that it caused their conflict, he would at times project from his own mind that his wife would always feel desirous/amorous for him even at inopportune times. She would say to him,

> that a woman, even in a relationship, marital or otherwise, has a right to say when, where, or how a sexual encounter may develop. The same goes for a man. Both have rights to make decisions as freely independent individuals.

The goal in this case was to minimally facilitate the husband to Stage 5, and perhaps to stimulate both of their development to Stage 6 moral judgment/reasoning. One incident stands out and typifies what became the fulcrum used with the Conceptual Template as a guide in fulfilling this goal. The incident occurred at an event where there was dancing.

The husband did not like dancing and was unwilling to dance with his wife; the wife danced with another man who was a friend of theirs. This was upsetting and later indicated to be unacceptable to the husband. In this instance, he became jealous and to some degree possessive. His wife found these emotional reactions to be unreasonable because she was "just having fun." She saw no harm in her behavior, and felt he was being unfair. He knew that she loved him, was committed to him and to their relationship. She liked to dance, whether with men or women, and thought it was fair, if he did not want to dance with her. There was the budding issue that she could not be herself, which denied her rights of self-identity, expression and autonomy as a person. These rights were common sense to her but were uncommon conventionally.

As earlier mentioned, her husband was self-reflective. He was interested in, and read books on self-improvement. As difficult as it was, he diligently worked to discover and apply what he was learning using the Conceptual Template as a model. He loved his wife and wanted to improve their relationship. When he discussed using the Conceptual Template in order to be more objective in his moral reasoning, he would sometimes comment that although being objective was difficult, it was good for their relationship and saw that it was fair even if he subjectively did not like it. He began to make the emotional connections necessary to become more empathetic to his wife's feelings or thoughts. He said that if he were in her position, he would feel the same way. Being free to make her choices independently was fair and just. He understood that he would want to be free to make his own choices, as did his wife, and she had every right, literally, to do so.

Being more objective, gave him insight that he had a right to choose. If he were to dance or not to dance his choice was independent of her will. Just as he had a right not to dance, she had a right to dance. Being more objective also made him more clearly see her commitment to him in her choices of dance partners, in respect to their relationship. He did not have to let jealousy come between them, as it was unfounded jealousy. He became aware that close friends of theirs also in committed relationships, sometimes danced with their friend's wives or husbands or both. He became grateful for their close friends dancing with her when he would not because she enjoyed it and it made her happy and there really was no issue for real jealousy to take control.

Both eventually developed to Stage 6 moral judgment/reasoning. The following are the three questions they were asked on follow-up a few years after marital counseling.

1. What was it like when you first learned the Conceptual Template (CT) process?
2. Was there a time when you thought the (CT) did not work but then it turned out that it did?
3. What is your outlook now with the (CT) as a resource?
4. What was it like when you first discovered the CT worked?

WIFE: When I went through the process of the CT, I felt like I was back in college and many of the ideas and "homework" challenges were something I had learned or done before. Once I realized how my level of moral development and thinking was different from my husband's level, yet both of us being capable of re-thinking on a higher level of moral development, I felt free. I felt my feelings were not only justified, but the entire functioning of my marriage was explainable and yet within this explanation was the hope to a better marriage. The initial excitement was also felt with a fear that my husband would not ever get there. He took much longer than me to see a new perspective.

On the lighter side, when a person finds out that the Conceptual Template works, it's like when you find out how changing your diet really works! You can exercise for hours a day, but it takes changing your diet to really make a difference on one's body. Much like equating this strategy to improving one's situation of despair by simply reading a "self-help" book, or going to a regular marriage counselor. A person can review events and regret or promise to change certain behaviors, but it isn't until one "thinks differently" that the real issues get resolved!

HUSBAND: When I first discovered that the Conceptual Template worked it was a new awareness that made my life so much easier as I didn't try to push everyone my way. It helped me in my marriage, relationship with my children and coworkers. I had and still have an everyday satisfaction and more hope for tomorrow.

Was there a time when you thought it didn't work but it turned out that it did?

WIFE: Perhaps a few times, in the beginning, I felt it working for me, but not for my husband, and I almost assumed that he just wasn't capable of reaching higher levels of thinking. Then later, after we stopped going to see Dr. Ries, when I would have a moment of thinking "Ugh, we are repeating the same ways"—well, when this occurred I would say to my husband, "Look, we can go back to the office and invite Dr. Ries to sit and hear our communication, but I need you to hear me without his presence. I need you to evaluate what I am saying as knowledge that is different from you and your current perspective. You must 'step away' from your one way of thinking, and really listen to what I am saying." Usually, at this point, the typical spiraling of misunderstandings and self-centered judgments halted, and my view was at least heard. One thing I liked about the CT was that it allowed both people to self-reflect on our own truths and verify our current values and aspirations for justice, but also we gained an understanding of our spouse's level of thinking, rationally or irrationally, and that too can be internalized to ask questions, verify and then make more sound judgments on any issue at hand.

HUSBAND: When I was introduced to the CT was during a marital crisis and I had, many times, when sex was involved, my animalistic side of me had a hard time to see what my wife valued and what was justice for her. But after thinking about CT, and as time went by I realized I wasn't thinking at a higher level.

What is your outlook now with the CT as a resource?

WIFE: I keep the chart on my fridge at all times. Guests stop in and say, "What is that?" I say, "It's the plan that is saving my marriage." When we finally got to the morality and justice criteria, Stage 6, I was empowered. I know that we both slip, I know that I process this CT faster and easier than my husband (a subjective thought), but I catch myself when I do or when he does. Once learned, it's difficult to return to the way of life we have been almost "programmed" to function and respond to. CT has lifted the enormous suffocation I was feeling within the typical "normal" marriage. I realize now that I don't walk around with suppressed feelings of "unjust" living with my husband and kids. I can separate myself from how they might be responding to events.

I understand that my independent nature does struggle within societies stereotypical concept of a wife and mother, but that I don't have to think of marriage this way. I don't have to behave and function within the lower levels of moral development. That I can be true to myself, my confident, independent self, and let my true being, my true personality, my true interests and desires to simply be exposed, yet not overlooked and viewed as anything less than equal.

I also have been the biggest advocate of the CT process and encouraged several of my friends to learn the template. Many who have gone for therapy, have made major changes to their lives, for the better!

HUSBAND: When I find myself in conflict I take a few minutes to stop and think and put the situation through the template and, believe it or not, it always comes out right for all parties because I'm now focused on cooperation. As a resource it is posted in our kitchen.

Summary and Conclusion

This chapter as the previous one focused on the implementation of the Conceptual Template with couples in which at least one individual was potentially transitioning from Conventional to Post-conventional moral reasoning. It was suggested that it was the female partner in both cases that appeared to have been, in part, affected by the events of the 1960s and 70s, either directly or indirectly. And further, it was suggested that this time period in our history was a catalyst of sorts in creating cognitive and cognitive-moral questioning/confusion particularly with respect to their social role identity eventually leading to the potential transition to Post-conventional moral judgment/reasoning.

Being aware of this potential transition or "what it looks like" is just as important as identifying stabilized stages, so as to be able to adjust the Conceptual Template dialogue with couples for both the understanding of the Conceptual Template process and also in order to facilitate moral development. In this regard, it is important for the practitioner when identifying couples stage(s) development and in order to facilitate development that individuals prefer the highest stage they comprehend, as referenced in the "characteristics or criteria of stages," specifically number

4 in Chapter 1. Further the prevalence of this potential transition in our society, namely, between Conventional and Post-conventional moral reasoning can be a common issue or concern when counseling couples. This quite dynamic potential transition is called moral relativism, which is, as earlier mentioned, an extreme form of moral subjectivism.

Chapter 6

Subjectivity and Objectivity
Moral Reasoning

Review

In the previous chapters, it has been implied or suggested, through the use of clinically based scenarios, that when couples develop in moral reasoning, there is parallel improvement in their relationships. According to Kohlberg (1984, p. 287), "Post-Conventional 'reasoners' tend to define norms in a much more similar fashion then do Pre- Conventional or Conventional 'reasoners'," appearing to suggest, to some degree, less conflict. The approach or method used with individuals who were engaged in couples therapy, was the implementation of the Conceptual Template model. The Conceptual Template facilitates moral reasoning through a process of conceptualizing and integrating essential philosophical concepts. The philosophical concepts integral and necessary for cognitive and cognitive-moral development, embodied in the Conceptual Template are: subjectivity, objectivity, truth, knowledge, belief/opinion, value, rights, morality and justice. The Conceptual Template is a representation of a natural process of reasoning discovered by the individual/couple through Socratic questioning. A Socratic method is used in order to elicit the meaning and interrelationships of these essential concepts/ideas, and when necessary, didactically refined, which then takes the form of the Conceptual Template. When conceptually integrated or understood, the resulting Conceptual Template awareness, can be consciously/mindfully applied to any experience in life, but more specifically and most importantly within the context of this book, to moral conflicts or experiences. Moral experiences are used here to connote how individuals/ couples treat one another especially in light of their moral reasoning in resolving conflicts of interests or claims. And, lastly, as it has been suggested, that it is the underlying moral reasoning or moral stages of cognitive development that parallel how couples interact and behaviorally treat one another (Kohlberg, 1981, Blasi, 1980).

Objective Reasoning

The Conceptual Template approach creates a conscious awareness or a mindfulness of essential concepts or ideas that the brain *naturally* uses to think/reason *objectively.* The faculty of reason can function for one, in consciously identifying or apprehending reality. And then, it is this faculty of cognition/reasoning that one uses to choose among viable options and how one can and will actually act or interact within the context of a particular reality in an ethically just manner. When the Conceptual Template is consciously applied it can lead to a greater awareness of *objective reasoning.* It can result in having greater objectivity about one's own subjectivity and that of others' subjectivity as well. And, it can thereby improve couples communication, understanding, transparency, trust, and intimacy with one another.

Objective and Subjective Reasoning

The conceptual awareness of objectivity or objective reasoning and being able to distinguish it from subjectivity or subjective reasoning, even if to only a limited degree, is indispensable to more fully understand our experiences. It is also the conceptual understanding and conscious awareness of the difference between these two specific ways of thinking that is critically important to not only logic and rational thought with regard to comprehending our experiences, but derivatively, to our interactional moral judgment/reasoning. Rational/judgment or reasoning and logic enable couples/individuals to also determine what is objectively and subjectively of value and/or of moral value when deciding on their actions as well as interactions with others, or in this context their significant other. The more adequately couples use objective reasoning in general, and objective-moral reasoning in particular, the better they are able to make judgments and decisions within the context of a given reality, and also to better understand their interpersonal interactions and choices. Being mindful of the difference between objective and subjective thinking then, whether in the non-moral or moral realm of human experience, can improve a couple's relationship and life together. It accomplishes this goal by making their life experiences both more intelligible and interpersonal interactions more equitable.

Objective and Subjective Modes of Reasoning/Cognition

When individuals or couples interpret the reality they are experiencing, whether it be personally or interpersonally, they can reason objectively, subjectively, or to some degree, a combination of both. Understanding the meaning of these essential concepts and being consciously aware of their meaning can significantly enhance couples' ability to resolve conflict. For example, a couple is in disagreement about which restaurant to visit to have dinner. One restaurant serves Italian food, the other American. Prices, ambiance and the like are similar. Nevertheless an argument ensues. The wife prefers the Italian restaurant. The husband the American food; he is a steak and potatoes man. They disagree as to which restaurant is "better." Being mindful of the meaning of subjectivity, it can be realized that which restaurant is "better" is purely subjective; either judgment is a preference and therefore personal. Therefore, there is not a rational or logical reason based upon reality to continue having conflict or being upset with one another because in this instance, "better," is purely *subjective*, that is, personal or *subject to only the mind of the beholder(s)*; it has nothing to do with reality per se. Another example is a disagreement occurs involving a couple, one of which is using an objective mode to support what is considered to be of value. The other is using a subjectively based mode of reasoning to support their opinion. It is again the conscious awareness of the difference in conceptual meaning or understanding of the modes being used, which would then logically and rationally lend itself, if applied, to resolution of the conflict. The conflict is, one individual has an opportunity to purchase a product that they have subjectively *wanted* (based upon personal reasons) for several years. However, objectively (based upon reality independent of personal wants), the cost is realistically exorbitant for this couple. If purchased, their mortgage could not possibly be paid. Being aware of each mode of thought, the wanted product, no matter how much and or how long desired is purely based upon a subjective mode of reasoning; it is therefore of subjective value or importance. The value of the mortgage payment, on the other hand, is derived from an objective mode of reasoning; it is based upon the reality in which they live. Being recognized as having objective value in contradistinction to a value that is subjectively based, would again rationally and logically resolve this dilemma. Objectively derived values, those based upon reality, would both logically and rationally supersede subjectively based values. In short, being unaware of the conceptual meaning of the mode being used in reasoning as in the above type of examples, can minimally result in confusion and/or conflict. Not having an awareness as to the conceptual meaning of these modes of cognition then, can result in mistaken reasoning. Ultimately, it is mistaken reasoning that can lead to the most severe problems and harmful consequences in human, or in this instance, couple interaction. This is particularly true in circumstances of moral conflict, or an issue involving what is fair or just. It is also an understanding and mindfulness of the conceptual meaning of these two essential modes of reasoning, that can lend itself to having less or diminished conflict. And, when conflict does occur, it can also provide a means for being more readily resolved.

The Importance of Definition and Meaning

Aristotle poignantly brought to our attention the monumental significance of definition and meaning for reasoning, understanding the nature of things, and communication in his following declaration.

If one were to say the word has an infinite number of meanings,
obviously reasoning would be impossible; for not to have one meaning
is to have no meaning, and if words have no meaning our reasoning
with one another, and indeed with ourselves, has been annihilated; for
it is impossible to think of anything if we do not think of one thing

(Aristotle, 1952)

Constructing Meaning through Objectivity

While both subjectivity and objectivity, can be beneficial or of value to our
lives, it is improvement in the development of objective thinking/reasoning
that can be a result of the Conceptual Template process that is critically
important in facilitating moral development and thereby also improve
couples' relationships (Ries 1979, 1981, 1992/2006). This begs the question
of "Why is understanding and being aware of objectivity or objective reasoning critical to moral development and/or to the improvement in
relationships?"

Objectivity or objective reasoning is critically, and most importantly,
salient, because it is this mode of reasoning, which we as humans use, in a
more or less adequate manner, in order to identify or conceptually construct the reality we experience. It is this objective process that, appre-
hends and identifies our sense perceptions, our interpretations, our
emotions and conceptualizations or our epistemological, metaphysical,
and meta-ethical constructs of reality. Therefore, it is also this process that
can bring to the foreground, the conscious awareness, mindfulness, or
identification of whether the process when being used interpersonally, in
the moral or non-moral domain, is itself being objective, subjective or a
combination of both. This understanding can then be objectively aligned
or realigned in order to understand the reality being considered individually or communicating with one another as a couple.

Human beings, as all living entities, appear to have a specific nature. It
is our specific human nature, through our faculty of reason, that mental
connections are formed. These mental connections, concepts, or construc-
tions are the "tools" of thought so to speak, or the means by which the
mind/brain is capable of discovering and/or identifying that which is
objectively true in reality. We do not survive through arbitrary means.
And, while from a scientific perspective it might be apparent that our
actions with regard to survival are not arbitrary, it is in the context of
moral reasoning, that it is not so apparent.

One possible explanation for the perception that moral judgment is
arbitrary or subjective might be gleaned from Kohlberg's description of
cognitive-moral development as occurring in an invariant sequence of
stages of "continual differentiation of moral universalizability from more

subjective ... beliefs" as stated above (1984, p. 283). And, while it *is* true that most people's moral reasoning is predominantly subjective as they are developing in their moral judgment/reasoning, the conclusion that is then often extrapolated from this experience is that all perception is subjective or relative (this will be discussed at length in the following Chapters 7 and 8 because of it saliency in moral development). This was earlier illustrated in Chapter 4 regarding the events of the 1960s and 70s. Because of a new found awareness that differing individuals, cultures or religions can have different ideas of what is morally "right" or "wrong" it was often concluded, therefore, "Who is any one person to say what is morally right or wrong, other than the individual, culture, or religion." This mistaken reasoning, is the philosophical idea of the "naturalistic fallacy" (Confusion of "is" with "ought") which can be or is resolved by development to Post-conventional moral judgment/reasoning. Post-conventional moral judgment/reasoning comprehends, for one, that because individuals may subjectively differ in their conceptualizations of what is beneficial, good, or just, does not mean that what is of moral value has no objective validity in fact. It means only that there is disagreement. Individuals and cultures made up of individuals can subjectively interpret reality differently; however, a reality is what it is, and that which is just in reality can in most instances be discovered or derived rationally and objectively in the nature of reality in which we all live. Our naturally occurring cognitive and cognitive-moral development is potentially capable of evolving into a universalizable and rational applicability of objective reasoning not only to our lives, or to the realities we experience, but objectivity is also essential with regard to the most adequate stages of moral development, that is, Post-conventional moral judgment/reasoning.

Operational Definitions of Objective and Subjective Reasoning

For the purpose here, objective reasoning and subjective reasoning can be operationally defined, as follows: Objective reasoning is the cognitive process of determining and proving what is true or false through identifying a correspondence or contradiction between thought, or a conceptual construct, and reality. It excludes that which exists solely in the mind's perception/interpretation when considering whether something is either true or false in reality. Said in another way, objective reasoning is focusing upon the attributes of the object, or characteristics, of the reality being considered; it excludes constructs of that which exists only in the mind when considering whether something is either true or false in reality.

Subjective reasoning, on the other hand, is deriving what one holds to be true or false upon one's personal or others of like mind's interpretation or constructs of the reality that is being considered. Or, said in another way, subjective reasoning is basing what one holds to be true or false on the subject's interpretation alone, or only upon emotional constructs or personal feelings, rather than upon the attributes of the reality being considered.

Subjectivity or subjective thinking then can be simply understood by couples as their own thinking; it is first and foremost, in a word, *personal*, or as stated earlier, *subject* to "the mind of the beholder." Subjectivity or subjective reasoning once understood by a couple can be didactically refined or defined by the practitioner, as one's own personal perspective, and that it is *only true* for one's self or those who are of like mind. To concretely support couples' understanding of subjectivity, the practitioner can didactically explain or give examples such as, that by definition, tastes, preferences, likes/dislikes, opinions and beliefs are all subjective constructs. And if necessary, or for additional clarification, it could also be said to couples, something both similar and as concrete as, that some people like the taste of chocolate ice cream, some prefer strawberry or vanilla, or some other flavor, all illustrate again subjective preferences. Further, it could be added that an individual might even assert a subjectively true statement with regard to their own preference, such as, one flavor is "better" than another, without realizing the subjectivity of their assertion. This assertion would only be true from their own perspective or others who subjectively have the same opinion; the truth or validity in subjective thinking only has a relation to one's own/personal interpretation of a reality; it has no direct relation or bearing to the truth or nature of things in respect to reality.

A classic example of this phenomenon's occurrence, namely subjectivity, both literally and figuratively, was considered so important to be understood, that it was illustrated in the "moral" of Socrates "story" in the book *Allegory of the Cave*; the prisoners in the cave believed their subjective perceptions or interpretations to be the reality. Another historical and clarifying example, which can be useful for the practitioner to discuss with couples in order to differentiate, and to further illuminate the importance of counterbalancing subjectivity with an understanding of objectivity, is the subjective idea or perception/interpretation of the earth being flat. Many people, at one time, believed the earth to be flat, and objectively this may still be the case for some people on this planet because it *visually* can appear to be so. This belief was based on the multitudes' visual experience. When they looked out onto the horizon it *appeared* flat as far as the eye could see. Not only did the earth or oceans, visually appear flat, it was also thought, or the forgone conclusion drawn by many people, was that when ships did not come back after going out to sea, they therefore "must have fallen over the edge of the flat earth." It was *subjectively* assumed that this was sufficient "proof" to then conclude that the earth was therefore, or must be, in fact, flat. This example also highlights the frequent mistaken subjective form of reasoning that draws conclusions, validation or acceptance of prevailing belief(s) or a subjective interpretations as being true simply because "authorities" or others think it is true or have agreed that it is true. Other more mundane examples that could be didactically used by a practitioner with couples in which people subjectively agree or find some form of validation of their personal interpretation of their experiences are found in clothing styles, fashion/statements, vehicles, speech patterns and even intonations. Those who are in the business of marketing products, often depend on this phenomenon or mistaken reasoning, namely, "perception is reality" to successfully sell products. For example, the mental association of people having fun at a party, and using a particular product, no matter the format, subjectively means or is perceived as, the product is enjoyable or has value, sometimes even if the product for some individuals is not normally of interest or was not previously associated with pleasure or value. The above types of subjective and concrete examples as well as others that are of a similar nature would usually or often be considered benign, with the possible exception of the earth being believed to be flat. We can imagine what life could be like having this belief. For example, on the lighter side, couples, who married during that time in human history might have chosen to forgo sailing on a ship to or for their celebratory honeymoon destination often to consummate their marriage. It is, however, in other forms of differing subjective opinions or beliefs, which are not or would not be considered lightly, particularly when it involves couples and, in general, human interaction that moral concerns can have serious consequences.

Subjective differences between couples can frequently cause conflict, elevate to heated disagreements, even harm, and become severely problematic. For example, individuals or couples having divergent moral beliefs or beliefs systems, some of which are or appear to be diametrically opposed, can create significant moral conflict. It is, especially relevant when beliefs or certain concrete values are subjectively misconstrued as being "objectively" of value. It can then be further believed and the conclusion reached, that others ought to agree or to adhere to these same "objective," actually subjectively based values. This can and has then been historically imposed on the actual objective inalienable rights of others, and can occur in a couple's relationship or interaction as well. As discussed earlier, of the expected "objective" social role identity, of women. Inherent in subjectivity, then, is perhaps the most important potential aspect of this form of reasoning. It is the mistaken idea/belief, again, that an experience(s) perception or interpretation of a reality is true, when it might or might not be true resulting in the forgone conclusion that because one subjectively perceives or interprets some experience to be true, it therefore is true. One significant missing element or underlying cause of this phenomenon, or mistaken reasoning, other than the above explanation of which Kohlberg has made us aware, namely, that the human mind naturally evolves from subjective thinking to being more objective, is not being consciously aware of the importance of questioning or adequately reflecting upon whether an interpretation of a particular reality is, in fact true.

The most common example of this mistaken type of reasoning is having and/or asserting an opinion/belief without an awareness of the necessity of substantive evidence or proof of its validity. I *believe* Socrates said: A wise wo/man is one who does not pretend to know that which they do not know. An opinion or belief does not constitute knowledge of a reality; *it is subject to doubt until objectively proven.* An opinion or belief therefore might or might not be true. Subjective reasoning, especially when unaware of one's own subjectivity or the subjectivity of one's partner when a couple is communicating their thought(s), can lead to misunderstanding and miscommunication. Whether aware of the importance of being mindful of our own and/or our partner's tendency toward subjectivity, it can nevertheless inadvertently result in confusion and conflict in the relationship.

Objective thinking/reasoning or objectivity, in contrast to subjective reasoning or subjectivity seeks to impartially understand a reality independent of one's personal subjective feelings, beliefs or opinions; it is based upon seeking substantive evidence or proof and thereby attempts to exclude, arbitrary predetermination, and forgone conclusions. It is, in a few words, a "disinterested pursuit of the truth." Therefore, for all intents and purposes, a construct that is based upon objective reasoning indicating a *proven* correspondence *between what is thought to be true and a reality constitutes knowledge of,* or an understanding of a reality (Socrates and/or Plato, Aristotle).

Human cognition, or thinking/reasoning then, is an underlying process of conceptual thoughts or ideas forming mental connections, resulting in constructs inferred from or directly from the reality that is experienced. As earlier mentioned, reasoning can be an objective process when, for example, identifying an actual reality, a subjective process when determining what we like, prefer or believe, and/or a combination of both when attempting to figure out what might be true in a given circumstance or reality. *Both modes can have value when understood and appropriately applied.*

As such, understanding the Conceptual Template approach to moral judgment/reasoning, in the context of being mindful of distinguishing these modes of reasoning, namely subjective, objective or a combination is salient. It is particularly important that this conscious awareness is being understood and used by the practitioner to specifically facilitate moral development. And, it is also important for couples to understand and have this mindfulness when using the Conceptual Template process in order to improve their communication, understanding, trust and intimacy with one another.

Summary and Conclusion

Objective and subjective thinking are operationally defined within the context of Aristotle's admonishment of the extreme importance of definition both in terms of constructing meaning in our reasoning as well as in our ability communicating with others. The importance of this understanding is then further delineated through examples of the underlying reasoning by which conflict arises when persons or couples do not understand these two essential modes of thought. It is then, that not being aware, whether because of cognitive development, lack of knowledge and/or not comprehending the difference between objectivity and subjectivity that the result can be mistaken reasoning which can then lead to misunderstandings, ranging from the benign to the most harmful interpersonal conflicts and consequences. The resolution of conflict whether in the moral or non-moral realms of human experience is the development of a conscious awareness/mindfulness of differentiating subjectivity from objectivity. The Conceptual Template approach to couple therapy creates a mindfulness of essential concepts the brain *naturally* has at its disposal to think/reason *objectively*. The understanding of the meaning or construct of objectivity as distinguished from subjectivity has the paralleling logical-rational realization; by definition, that subjectivity flows in the wake of objectivity in being solely personal. The consequences of conflating these extremely critical terms magnifies Aristotle's *admonishment* to all of us in respect of the importance of understanding the meaning of words and the value of these specific words/constructs, both in the non-moral and moral realms of human experience, or in this context, the interpersonal experiences of couples.

Chapter 7

Cognition

Subjectivity and/or Relativity and Objectivity

Cognition can be understood in terms of it being the underlying mental processing for our understanding of information from our experiences. This process as suggested in Chapter 6, can be predominantly objective, subjective or used in combination. As such, cognition or our thinking/underlying reasoning both directly affects and indirectly influences our moral reasoning. Stated in cognitive developmental terms, moral stages have an underlying cognitive component. Piaget discussed this as "horizontal decalage" in which there is a generalization of cognitive developmental stages to other areas of development, such as, in this instance, moral development (Kohlberg, 1981, p. 92). However, while cognitive development is necessary for moral development, it is not a sufficient condition (Kohlberg, personal communication) (also Kohlberg, 1981, p. 92). In other words, a person could be highly developed cognitively yet nevertheless be undeveloped in their moral reasoning. For example, an individual who is the president of a large corporation, which would suggest being highly developed in their cognition because otherwise they could not succeed in this position of oversight, could in their moral reasoning operate at the Pre-conventional level. Further, whether we are either predominantly subjective or predominantly objective in our cognition in a particular domain, such as at work, our moral reasoning can differ depending on the domain. Or again, to say in another way, cognition is the underlying process for both subjective and objective forms of reasoning, whether it is in the non-moral or moral realm of human experience.

Objective Reasoning

In the non-moral realm, a person can use predominantly objective reasoning in their work, such as doing scientific research or making sure widgets are attached correctly, and nevertheless be subjective in their social/interpersonal interaction with others, such as their spouse and other members in a family. Or in the moral realm, a person whose social role identity is a Supreme Court judge, could be at the most adequate stage of moral development Post-conventional Stage 5 or 6. At this level of development they could be capable of making objective Post-conventional legal deci-sions that affect society. They might, however, use subjective Conventional moral Stage 3 and/or 4 reasoning in other areas of social/interpersonal life. For example, being rule oriented (Stage 4) in their Conventional social role identity with significant others as a mother, nurturer, or as a father, provider. It is then, that a person can reason differently from one domain to the next. Reasoning can be effected by other variables, includ-ing and specifically a particular domain, the issue being considered, and even one's social role identity, (Ries, 1979, 1981, 1992/2006). And, it is also the case that either subjective or objective reasoning, whether in the non-moral or moral realm can also be consistent across domains. Being consistently subjective across domains appears most common; however, it does not appear to be uncommon for people having some level of objec-tivity in one domain to not be consistent in this form of reasoning across domains, as indicated. Further, even with clearly understood objectivity or objective reasoning there can be an element of subjectivity. At the Post-conventional Stage 5, there can be more than one perspective that is based upon objective reasoning or having an objective basis. This is precisely what Post-conventional Stage 6 resolves. By constructing a principle that meets the criteria of reversibility and universaliability an objective princi-ple can be agreed upon by all concerned, including the least advantaged, as fair or just even if there is *subjective disagreement*.

Subjective Reasoning

When subjective reasoning occurs with respect to a reality that is, in fact, purely a subjective experience, such as about what is liked, preferred, one's personal beliefs, opinions, and so on, it is not in itself cognitively contra-dictory. When it is believed to be contradictory by another or others sub-jective opinion(s), this is when conflict can arise, within a person's own subjectivity or the subjectivity of another or others. It does not necessarily create cognitive conflict or contradiction within one's own cognitive pro-cesses, or for that matter, have any significant consequence, that is, when a person is aware that their thinking, or that of others is, subjective. Rhetori-cally, it might be asked: "*Why would it?*" Likes, dislikes, tastes, preferences, opinions and beliefs are all, by definition or meaning, subjectively/personally true, pure and simple. There is no degree of objectivity that could lead one to find contradiction in one's own subjectivity, or that of others regarding sub-jective matters, that is, and once again, if one is cognizant of the meaning of subjectivity or is mindful of its meaning and relevance to our personal experiences of reality. It is, however, to reiterate, if a person does not have an understanding of the meaning of subjectivity and they think that their sub-jectivity or perception is the truth, no matter what the circumstances might be, it is then, that it can lead to conflict with more or less serious consequences. It could, for example, lead to a couple having an argument over something purely subjective, which could then lead to even greater consequences particularly if both think they are correct and believe that they are being "objective" with respect to their subjective perception regarding a reality. Or conversely, as earlier suggested in Chapter 6, being consciously aware of what subjectivity means or is, it then should not result in any conflict at all; it is after all subjective. Again, "Why would it?" There is no inherent conflict in subjectivity, it is personal, and it has nothing to do with truth or reality other than to the person who experiences something in a personal way.

For example, a couple is going out to dinner and just before leaving home one asks the other the subjective question, "How does what I am wearing look?" and the other responds by saying, without malevolent intent, "You look horrible in that outfit!" thinking that what they are expressing subjectively is, in reality or in fact, true. If both understand subjectivity and realize it is merely an opinion or it is expressed that in their opinion they do not personally like how it looks, then perhaps the consequences of the earlier mentioned response would be mitigated. If they realize or are mindful of what subjectivity is, they can then respond in numerous ways consistent with objectivity of their own subjectivity or their partner's, and that would be, or allow for, a more intimate form of acceptance, communication or understanding of their significant other's mind and vice versa. The response to the initial question could have been: "Do you like or feel comfortable with what you are wearing?" perhaps adding, with the realization of subjectivity "I think you are attractive no matter what you wear: You are beautiful naked." When individuals reason subjectively about their experiences because of not understanding what subjective reasoning is as distinguished from objective reasoning, they tend to generalize this form of thinking, when interpreting reality The result can therefore be that the individual cannot fathom that what they subjectively interpret their perception to be, with respect to a reality that is experienced, would be anything else but as they perceive or believe it to be. They believe what they think is true, when in fact, it might or might not be true. It is not dissimilar to a child who has not yet reached object permanence. Because something is no longer seen, "it, no longer exists." Until the child or the adults begin questioning their own as well as others reasoning or conclusions, subjectivity blankets the mind.

Another reason for the phenomenon of subjective reasoning being generalized across domains, for example, subjective cognition leading to subjective moral judgment/reasoning, is the naturally occurring underpinning invariant sequence of cognitive development, as well as cognitive-moral development. As stated earlier, at the beginning of development, stages begin as purely subjective, and then, over time, as development occurs, there is the potential for further differentiation toward a greater degree of objective reasoning with respect to reality. Or, with regard to moralization, as indicated in Chapter 6, "Our research shows that individual development in moral reasoning is a continual differentiation of moral universalizability from more subjective ... beliefs" (Kohlberg, 1984, p. 283). It appears, that this phenomenon, at least, in part, is a significant component of both cognitive and cognitive-moral development, and as also earlier mentioned, horizontal decalage. Even though a natural occurring aspect of human development, this phenomenon can nevertheless be problematic. It can cognitively blind us from understanding a given reality, which can affect couples' interaction and relationship with regard to understanding of one another, and therefore their communication and intimacy.

At the extreme, for couples or for others, not understanding what subjective reasoning is, or when it takes the form of mistaken reasoning, it can individually and interactively potentially cause even life-threatening consequences. This phenomenon of the generalization of subjective reasoning can be of a serious matter not only in the non-moral domain as implied and discussed; it is also the case, in causing conflict in human interactions in general and in couples' relationships. All of the above when viewed from the perspective of the moral domain is the subject matter of the phenomenon of moral subjectivism and/or relativism and reflects the importance of specifically facilitating moral development.

The practitioner understanding of this phenomenon, even if only in part, for intervening in this naturally occurring process of moralization at an appropriate time period developmentally, that is, in order to facilitate moral development, which might not otherwise spontaneously occur, can be of significant value. Lastly, cognitive conflict, even if the individual is not consciously aware of inherent contradiction or it is not consciously reflected upon, appears necessary for both cognitive and cognitive-moral development. But, again to reiterate, "Why would a person question their thinking if they do not in some conscious way objectively recognize the inherent contradiction in their thinking or reasoning as manifested, for one, in moral subjectivism/relativism?" Perhaps it is the critical importance of this phenomenon that is the reason some of the greatest thinkers discussed this contradictory form of reasoning.

Subjectivism and Relativism

The subject matter of subjectivism and relativism is not new. And, these modes of reasoning are as important or significant today as they were since the dawn of humanity or human interaction. As early as the fifth century BC, Protagoras, the Greek sophist, posited, according to Socrates, in Plato's Theaetetus, the "...argument in which all things are said to be relative, in the dictum, Man is the measure of all things...." Socrates summarizes the Protagoras argument in Plato's *Theaetetus* (1952, p. 522), saying, "...that whether a person says that a thing is or becomes, he must say that it is or becomes to or of or in relation to something else; but he must not say…that anything is or becomes absolutely." Socrates concludes "I wonder that he did not begin his book on Truth with a declaration that a pig or a dog-faced baboon…is the measure of all things." Centuries later, Shakespeare expressed what could be interpreted as the essence of a morally subjective/relativistic orientation when he has Hamlet say: "…for there is nothing either good or, bad but thinking makes it so" (Shakespeare, 1947, p. 63). Spinoza again echoed this ethically subjective/relativistic view saying "…one and the same thing might at the same time be both good and evil or indifferent." Aristotle (1954, p. 525), also aware of this idea declares, "It is impossible for the same man at the same time to believe the same thing to be and not to be…."

In more recent times, these ideas are used in connection to ethical reasoning. Brandt (1959) suggests that ethical relativism can be defined in the following manner.

> There are conflicting ethical opinions that are equally valid…that one ethical statement cannot be shown 'objectively' to be more valid than another…that either there is no unique rational method or justified method in ethics, or that the use of the unique rational method in ethics, in the presence of an ideally complete system of factual knowledge would still not enable us to make a distinction between the ethical statements being considered.
>
> (Brandt, 1959, pp. 273–266)

Frankena (1963, pp. 92–93) similarly summarizes the relativist position:

> It holds in the basic ethical or value judgment there is no objectively valid rational way of justifying one against another; consequently, two conflicting basic judgments may be equally valid.

Relativism, according to Kohlberg (1970s), as a number of his student asserted is:

> A questioning of the validity of … One's ability to make moral judgments about or for others or for others to make moral judgments applicable to oneself.
> …there are no such things as valid moral principles, no objective sense in which one thing is morally better than another.
>
> (Kohlberg and Gilligan, 1971)

Further, Turiel (1972, p. 13) suggests that: Individuals who express three of the following four following criteria or characteristics are considered to be morally relativistic.

1. All values are relative and arbitrary.
2. One should not judge what another person should do.
3. It is up to every individual to make his/her own decisions.
4. Terms like duty, good, should, or moral have no meaning.

Fishkin (1976) in his study of relativism suggests that definitions such as the aforementioned, conflate into a single category various forms of this psychological phenomenon. This is due, according to Fishkin, "...to emphasis having been placed upon analysis of normative moral judgments, with respect to first order questions of prescriptions for moral action (in particular cases or in general cases of actions), rather than upon meta-ethical reasoning that concerns second order questions, or the basis for such 'first order' assertions."

Fishkin delineates four positions of meta-ethical relativism. They are "relativism," subjectivism, personalism, and amoralism. Fishkin brings to light, specific differentiating characteristic of this phenomenon, which are important to both those involved in research regarding this psychological phenomenon or to those who would value a more in-depth understanding of this phenomenon. Kohlberg found value in Fishkin distinguishing four positions of meta-ethical relativism such that the term moral relativism was later used interchangeably with moral subjectivism or radical subjectivism in light of Fishkin's research. Kohlberg in a later discussion of relativism, namely, in his monumental book, *The Psychology of Moral Development* (1984, Vol. II), uses the terms relativism and subjectivism interchangeably. And further, he suggests in light of Fishkin's refinement of this relativistic phenomenon, terms such as "radically 'subjectivistic'" or "'radical subjectivism'" or "extreme relativism." However, when personally doing research regarding relativism, from 1974–1981, "relativism" was the term used by Kohlberg and in Kohlberg's and Turiel's research in regard to this phenomenon as a potential transition to Post-conventional moral judgment/reasoning. In his book (1984), Kohlberg continued to re-define, re-fine, and use the terms subjectivism and/or relativism interchangeably. It is in this later refinement that he also appears to represent relativism, using terms such as "radical relativism" or "radically subjectivistic" interchangeably.

For clinical purposes, these distinctions are important only in so far as they distinguish the more extreme form of relativism, where an absolutistic and dogmatic stance is taken from the less extreme forms of either subjectivism or relativism that is most common in society. These issues will be further addressed in Chapters 8.

Summary and Conclusion

Cognition is defined as the underlying mental process of thinking or reasoning in comprehending our experiences. This faculty or ability of forming mental connections from sense perceptions to forming conceptualization or constructs occurs in a manner that is subjective, objective or a combination of both. While this faculty may be likened to neurological conduit specifically of reasoning itself, it also provides, in this context, the underpinnings or basis for moral reasoning; Piaget used the term "horizontal decalage" to describe and explain that reasoning is an ability that is used, influences, generalized, effects and therefore *parallels* other areas of cognition. To illustrate this process in cognitive-moral developmental terms, cognitive development is a *necessary condition* but not a sufficient *condition* for moral development (Kohlberg, personal communication). Or similarly, the most adequate stages of moral reasoning require formal operational reasoning, although formal operational thought alone is not sufficient for the most adequate stage of moral reasoning; an individual can be highly developed cognitively yet undeveloped in their moral reasoning. While there is horizontal decalage of the reasoning process itself that effects, or parallels other domains of cognition, it is not necessarily a one-to-one relationship.

Given that objective, subjective, or a combination are modes of cognition or reasoning, they too affect the constructs formed in other domains. Examples are given to demonstrate these differing modes in other domains, however, for our purpose it is in the moral domain that is of interest, particularly with regard to *moral subjectivity* and its more extreme form of *moral relativity*, which subvert, in a manner of speaking, the human potential for reasoning more objectively about moral issues and development to Post-conventional moral judgment/reasoning.

The subject matter and the psychological phenomena moral subjectivity and relativity are not new. Through the words of great thinkers as far back in history as the fifth century BC the phenomena of subjectivity and its more extreme form, relativism, are found in literature and philosophy and are quoted. More recent researchers, most notably Kohlberg as well as other knowledgeable individuals defining these terms in relation to objectivity are discussed, to more clearly differentiate or tease out their meaning so that the practitioner can align this approach to facilitate moral development.

Each of these modes of cognition has value when understood and appropriately applied. It is however when these modes are not clearly differentiated, or there is a lack of awareness of the inherent subjective contradictions that can cognitively occur, that it can lead to unabated confusion and conflict mistaken reasoning. In a sense this event is moral subjectivity and relativity "writ large." Subjective interpretation is then deemed to be reality; everything is subjective or relative, including morality. The conclusion emanating from moral subjectivity and relativity is that there is then no objective means of determining what is fair or just in the resolution of conflicting claims.

Resolving contradictions/confusion, specifically in moral reasoning is the goal of Conceptual Template and can lead to Post-conventional moral reasoning. Kohlberg and Turiel then, were correct in their hypothesis that moral "relativism" is a potential transition to a Post-conventional moral orientation. And, it is the facilitation of development of moral reasoning, manifested behaviorally in couples treating one another in a just manner, or respecting each other's dignity, that can provide the foundation for trust, transparency, and intimacy, ultimately improving the couples' interpersonal interaction.

Chapter 8

Clinically Identifying Moral Subjectivism/Relativism through Implementing Moral Dilemmas

This chapter's definition of relativism as distinguished from subjectivism is based upon earlier research (Ries, 1979, 1981, 1992/2006) as well as later clinical observations (1981–present). Understanding this information in order to determine whether the individual(s) or couple is subjective in their moral reasoning or is reasoning in the more extreme form of subjectivism, namely moral relativism, allows the counselor to more clearly identify a couple's placement within the framework of Kohlberg's developmental stages. Clinically determining, both prior to and at the end of the Conceptual Template counseling process whether an individual or couple is, subjective, relativistic, or objective in their moral reasoning is a valuable measure. It can be used to identify status and/or placement of the individual/couple in respect to Kohlberg's invariant sequence of moral stages. Also, understanding this distinction will allow the practitioner to have a clearer perspective in the use of the Socratic method in the Conceptual Template process of questioning couples in order to elicit the essential concepts, their meaning and interrelationship.

Moral subjectivism, and moral relativism, for the purpose here, will be *clinically* described or defined with consideration of historical philosophical meanings, psychological definitions based upon and for research, and redefining and refining in order to bring greater clarity in its clinical application. With this understanding then, and for the purpose of clinical identification, *moral subjectivism* is the germinal construction of what can potentially lead to its more extreme form, namely, *moral relativism*.

Moral Subjectivism

Individuals having become aware of the actual ubiquitous existence of subjective morality, whether it be with respect to other individuals, religions or cultures having different ideas of what is considered morally right or wrong, results in the conclusion that morality is purely subjective. This is the philosophical idea of the Naturalistic Fallacy of confusing "Is" and "Ought." This fallacy lacks the awareness that just because something is, exists or occurs, for example in another society, does not mean that is the way it should/ought to be, or is morally just. Although defined in various ways, essentially the moral subjectivist for our clinical purposes holds that moral value is based on one's own beliefs/opinions or, in other words, is *relative* to the individual, a particular group, culture or religion. In short, morality or that which is morally valued in this context is considered to be, in a word, *personal*. The moral subjectivist's construct of morality being personal or subjective, leads to the erroneous conclusion that, therefore, that which is moral can *only be determined for one's self* or relative to the self, and therefore cannot and should not be made for any other person, culture, or religion. Morality then is considered to be independent of the objective conditions or the nature of any given reality.

Moral Relativism

Moral relativism is clinically defined here for operational purposes as a more radical form of subjectivism. Like subjectivism, in which the individual has recognized the prevalent existence of subjective morality, it results in a more extreme form of subjectivism. This is because the cognitive differentiation has not yet developed sufficiently to resolve this potentially perplexing subjective condition, that it can lead over time to a different and more extreme form of an erroneous conclusion. There is no *objective* way to determine what is morally right or wrong.

This manner in which subjective reasoning is distinguished from relativistic thinking is, in this context, for the purpose of clinical identification or application. In order to clinically identify moral subjectivity and relativism, a couple can be asked individually or separately. This can be done using either a paper and pen or individual session to avoid being influenced by one's significant other to respond to one of the following three moral dilemmas.

Note: It is the underlying reasoning of a response not the content that indicates stage assignment(s).

Slavery Dilemma

Let us say that, in one culture their laws, culture, traditions, beliefs permit slavery and therefore they have slavery. And, let's say that, in another culture their laws, culture, traditions, beliefs, and so on do not permit slavery, and therefore they do not have slavery. Is one culture right and the other one wrong, or are they equally right? Why?

Subjective Moral Reasoning

Clinically, a morally subjective response to the slavery dilemma, as in this actual example would typically include the following elements,

Personally, I think the culture that has slavery is morally wrong, but then, I am from a different culture. I also have different religious beliefs, so I cannot judge someone who has different religious beliefs. Laws (Stage 4) may differ between country, culture and/or religion; therefore, I cannot say what is right or what is wrong for them. What is morally right or wrong for anyone else who has different beliefs is personal or individual.

A practitioner would then ask, to determine or clarify whether the individual is subjective, "Are you morally right and they are wrong, or are you both equally right?" The typical responses of the client(s) are as follows for the moral subjectivist.

I can't say what is morally right or wrong for another culture? I can't say what is right or wrong for anyone else. I can't say what is right for them. I can only say what is morally right for me.

A practitioner may further probe by asking again, "Is one culture right and the other wrong or are they equally right?" An individual who is morally subjective in their reasoning will inevitably say, "We are equally right." These responses are clinically indicative of the psychological phenomenon of moral subjectivism.

Morally subjective reasoning specifically at the Conventional Level, Stages 3 and/or 4 will say what they personally believe to be morally right or wrong, however, they nevertheless think that morality is personal or subjective. Further they will reason that they do not have a "right" to say what is morally right or wrong for anyone else because it is to them that morality is subjective. The resulting conclusion of morally subjective reasoning, even in opposing moral judgments, is that they are considered to be *equally valid*. Individuals who are morally subjective do not understand or realize the contradiction or mistaken reasoning in this logic. The contradiction in ethical reasoning within this moral dilemma, and the reasoning held by the moral subjectivist in order to resolve and/or determine the individual's choice or action, is, a logical contradiction, in that, it cannot both be right and wrong at the same time, if polar opposites under the same circumstances. Said in another way, something is either morally right or wrong, something cannot both be and not be at the same time as Aristotle so eloquently said: "The same man at the same time cannot ... believe something to be and not be" (Aristotle, 1952, p. 525).

Further, the morally subjective individual does not realize the contradiction in their subjectivity of it is up to each individual to decide what is morally right or wrong for themselves, in that it is against the will of the individuals who are enslaved, it is not up to them, they have no choice.

How then can everyone else's subjective decision, be of equal value when it affects others?

Relativistic Moral Judgment

Regarding probing clients in order to determine if there is a clinical quality of the morally relativistic phenomenon occurring in their moral judgment/reasoning, the practitioner may use a moral dilemma, again such as the slavery dilemma, and inquire how the client would respond. The following responses would indicate morally relativistic reasoning. "There is no such thing as morally right or wrong." or "Good and bad have no meaning," or "They are both wrong" the latter of which when probed will reflect the former responses in various ways. And, less common, "Whatever they choose to do, or choose not to do, it is not up to anyone else to say what anyone else should or should not do, as *should has no meaning.*" The moral relativist might even say, and has said, "Whether they have slavery or not is arbitrary. It is all relative."

Post-conventional Moral Reasoning/Judgment

At the Post-conventional level of moral reasoning, there would be no evidence of subjectivity/relativity but rather there would be an objective response to the slavery dilemma, that slavery is unjust with the following reasoning. The reasoning underlying their response would be that slavery is denying the individuals freedom or liberty, or their right to freedom, or the slave is being treated as if they are the property of another when they are a person and therefore slavery is morally wrong. The following are typical responses at the Post-conventional level of moral reasoning.

> It is wrong to have slavery. Regardless of the culture's belief or laws; slavery is denying that person(s) human right of freedom. It is denying that person(s)freedom to make their own choices. The culture that has slavery is morally wrong because they are treating human beings as property. The slaves are human beings, not property, even if believed to be or legally defined that way.

The practitioner may use the following question to probe even further, to confirm Post-conventional, moral, objective reasoning rather than subjectivism.

> Even though you think it is morally wrong to have slavery, does that make it morally wrong? If others think differently, that slavery is morally right in their culture would you be *equally right* or would one culture be right and the other wrong?

The following are typical responses at the Post-conventional level of moral reasoning.

> No, we are not equally right. What they are doing is not a matter of opinion. It is a matter of human rights, of which we are all entitled. They are wrong because they are not respecting the slaves' human rights or their dignity (Kohlberg, personal communication).

The purpose of determining moral subjectivism or relativism using the **Heinz dilemma** instead or in addition to the slavery dilemma can be to more clearly highlight the underlying thought process or structure and the corresponding predominant moral stage(s). The Defining Issue Test (DIT) could also be expediently used for this purpose (Rest, 1979). It can be scored at the University of Alabama, Center for Ethical Development. The Standard Form-Issue Scoring Manual developed at the Center for Moral Education at Harvard University requires extensive training.

Heinz Dilemma

In Europe, a woman was near death from a special kind of cancer. There was one drug that the doctors thought might save her. It was a form of radium that a druggist in the same town had recently discovered. The drug was expensive to make, but the druggist was charging ten times what the drug cost him to make. He paid $400.00 for the radium and charged $4,000.00 for a small dose of the drug. The sick woman's husband, Heinz, went to everyone he knew to borrow the money and tried every legal means, but only could get together $2,000.00, which is half of what it cost. He told the druggist that his wife was dying, and asked him to sell it cheaper or let him pay later. But the druggist said, "No I discovered the drug and I'm going to make money from it." So, having tried every legal means, Heinz gets desperate and considers breaking into the man's store to steal the drug for his wife. Should Heinz steal the drug? Why or why not?

Why is it right or wrong? Is it actually right or wrong whether or not Heinz steals the drug? Or, if someone else disagrees with what you think, are you right and they are wrong or are you/they equally right?

Subjective Thinking at Conventional Stage 3

The practitioner may probe the individual with the following question to the Heinz dilemma to preliminarily identify the predominant stage of moral reasoning. "Should Heinz steal the drug?" The following responses would be indicative of Stage 3 moral reasoning, "Yes, because *life is sacred*. Yes, *he loves his wife, so he should save her.*"

The following are a few questions the practitioner may ask to probe further in order to confirm the corresponding phenomena of moral subjectivism. "What if he doesn't love his wife? What if he doesn't think life is sacred? Should he still steal the drug in order to save her life even if he doesn't love his wife or even if he doesn't think that life is sacred?" Moral subjectivism would be indicated in Stage 3 subjective responses such as if it were then stated, "Well why would he save her *if he doesn't love her?*" Or, "He should save her anyway: they are still married." Other typical Conventional Stage 3 responses indicating subjectivity are: "Yes, if he *loves* her. I probably would because it would be *my wife and I love her.*" Or, "I would have stolen the drug *because life is precious* and you can't put a price on it because *he should care about her or love her. H*e shouldn't just sit back and let her die."

If then asked, "If someone thought different then you, for example, they think it would be wrong to steal the drug even though Heinz loved and cared about his wife, would he be wrong?" An actual response for this example, "It is up to the person, *how much* they love their wife or not." "I think it would be more likely that the *closer* a husband feels toward his wife, the more likely he would steal the drug, but I don't think that being very close to the wife would necessarily obligate him to steal the drug or vice versa." Later this same individual said, "I have been doing some thinking on this and *I have to take both sides. I couldn't begrudge him either way.*"

Subjective Thinking at Conventional Stage 4

At Stage 4, responses to, "Should Heinz steal the drug for his wife?" indicating typical subjectivity are: "No, he shouldn't steal, it is *illegal,* but *personally* I would probably steal it." And, when then asked, "why?" or the reason he should not, or he should, steal the drug, the responses could be a number of personally held beliefs or convictions, such as "It is *against the law*" or "It is against my *religious beliefs,* 'Thou shalt not steal'" to mention a few Stage 4 responses. Or, more typically the response is "Yes, I think Heinz should steal the drug for his wife." But when then asked "Why? Or what is the reason Heinz should steal the drug for his wife, there can be a number of differing personal/subjective, responses such as "He *should because the law* is too general and isn't taking into account the circumstances in this case." Or "*Laws* don't work in every case, they're sometimes to specific or rigid in some ways." "A lot of times laws like this can't be applied in all situations. Sometimes they're too limited." "He should, *because God's law is* more important." And, when asked. "Is it actually right or wrong?" the response would be subjectively stated by responding for example, "Well, I don't think he should steal, but somebody might not believe the way I do and think he or she should steal the drug." And if further probed, by asking "Are you right and they wrong, or are you equally right," they will say, "Equally right," and if asked to justify this response they will respond by saying, for example, "I can only say what would be right for me, I can't say what is right for someone else." And, if further probed as to whether they are right and the other person wrong, their response would again indicate it's a personal/subjective decision, such as, "It is up to them, I cannot say what they should do."

Relativistic Thinking

If experiencing the more extreme form of subjectivism, namely, relativism, the individual would respond to stealing the drug by saying such things as, "I can't say that my decision is morally right, I would save my wife because *I love her* and I don't want her to die. *It has nothing to do with morality. I am not sure there is such a thing.*" "Or laws have nothing to with morality even if they maintain some form of social order. Laws are just to make people do what others want them to do and to believe they need laws. It is just what people want to believe." "Different religions governments, and people have different beliefs. *"So how can there be right or wrong, it is all relative."*

Post-conventional Thinking

At the Post-conventional level of moral reasoning the responses would be objective by recognizing in this instance, that the issue of life has a greater value than property. It would be taken into consideration that there is to some degree a *hierarchy of values*, such as objective derived values are more important than subjective based values. Also the Post-conventional individual would understand rights, namely, that which people are entitled to by virtue of their existence, and are thereby objectively derived from reality or appertain to humans' right to existence.

> He should steal the drug if he has no other recourse. The druggist has a right to his property, but the wife also has a right to her life. They both are objective values in reality, but a human life or a person's right to life, although, unfortunate in this instance from the perspective of the druggist, would nevertheless supersede his right to his property.

(Hierarchy in terms of objectively derived values). Or,

> I think that he should steal the drug to save his wife. The druggist's right to his property would not exist without human life that determines what is of value for our lives whether it be the druggist or the wife or Heinz.

Objectively, we would all think our life is more important in this situation. "The druggist is being subjective in his decision to not give Heinz the drug, and then he should be paid later?" Or,

> He should steal the drug to save his wife's life even though it is against the law. The law should protect peoples' rights. In this case the law isn't, it is infringing on the right from which all other rights are based, even the druggist having a right to his drug. But the law is infringing on Heinz's wife's right to her life.

"Without life there would not be rights. Not even the druggist would have a right to his drug or his property. 'Yeah,' he should definitely steal the drug."

If then asked, for determining any form of subjectivity, even relativity, "if someone else thought that Heinz should not steal the drug for his wife because it is against the law, would you think they are wrong or would you be equally right?"

> They would be wrong, because they would not be understanding that the law in Heinz's wife's circumstances is denying her right to live, it is actually doing just the opposite, it is infringing or her right, her right to life.

Chicken Bone Dilemma

A group of friends were celebrating Tom's birthday. Tom was eating and began to laugh when a bone from a chicken wing suddenly was drawn into his throat and he began to choke. His friends are unable to dislodge the chicken bone and are concerned that an ambulance would have difficulty finding the house due to its location. They decide that driving to the hospital is his best chance for survival, nearly 10 minutes away, if there is no traffic.

Between 30–180 seconds of oxygen deprivation, a person may lose consciousness At the one-minute mark, the brain cells begin dying. At three minutes, neurons suffer more extensive damage, and lasting brain damage becomes more likely. At five minutes, death becomes imminent. At 10 minutes, even if the brain remains alive, a coma and lasting brain damage are almost inevitable. At 15 minutes, survival becomes nearly impossible.

As they were taking Tom to the hospital, there was a traffic light at the bottom of the mountain and it turned red. The hospital was not far away but if they stopped at the red light and waited for it to turn green they thought he would most likely die.

Facing a red light, with Tom choking to death in the backseat and the hospital looming ahead, should the driver run the red light?

Why or why not?

What is your reasoning?

What exactly would you do?

If one of Tom's friends would choose to run the red light and the other would not, is one right and the other wrong or are they equally right?

Stage 3 Subjective Moral Reasoning

In the chicken bone dilemma, responses to the question "What should they do?" A person who is Stage 3 using subjective reasoning could say, "He should run the red light because he is their *friend,* and *that's what friends are for, to be there for you at times when you really need them.*" Or, "They should run the red light because they are *good friends* and really ... *care about him, or* why would they go along racing to the hospital." If then asked, "What if someone said that they did not think they should run the red light," for example, "No they shouldn't run the red light, because they could get in an accident and maybe *hurt* somebody, maybe somebody they even know and like...And then they would probably *feel real guilty.*"

If then asked, "would you be right and they are wrong, or would you be equally right?"

Well, of course I think I'm right for the reasons I said, but someone else might have different reasons, like the person being worried about hitting another car and being in an accident. It is really up to the person. They have a 'right' to do what they think they should do. *Maybe they aren't that good of friends (Stage 3)* with Tom, the person choking. *It is really up to them what they do.*

If then probed further, and asked, "You said that you think you are right even though someone else might not think the same way as you do." If then asked, "Are you actually right and they are wrong or are you equally right?" *We are equally right.* I can't tell someone else what is right or wrong for him or her. I can only say what I think I should do, and I believe that *friends or people who care* about each other should do everything they can to *help* each other." Conversely, it is also possible, as just indicated, that someone who is at Conventional Stage 3, would say, "He should not run the red light" for reasons such as, "Others will understand why we didn't run the light even if Tom didn't survive." Or from a religious perspective at Stage 3 a person might say, "No he shouldn't run the red light, I believe that God will make sure that everything will work out for the best." Or, "no, *Tom would understand* that it is not right to run the light and so would his parents and *I am a good person* just *following my conscience.*"

If then asked, "Others asked this same question disagree with you. They think just the opposite of you. They think they should run the red light.

Are you actually right and they are wrong or are you equally right?" Again, a Stage 3 subjective response would be, "We are *equally right*." It is up to whatever the person believes is right, and I can't make a judgment on what they believe is right anymore than they can make a decision of what I believe or should do."

Stage 4 Moral Reasoning

At Stage 4, responses to the question "Should they run the red light" could be, "No, they should not run the red light; *it is against the law*." "Or no he should not run the light someone else in another car could be coming the other way and they get killed. If people did that there would be a lot of accidents and a lot of people would get hurt or killed." "*That is why we have laws*." If further probed by asking them, "Well it is your friend or someone you care about and you are trying to help, so why wouldn't you run the light."

> The traffic light is for everyone, to protect us, that is why we have them. I agree that I would rather run the light because it is my friend, and I would probably feel real guilty about it, but the law is specific and maybe too limiting, but we still need to obey laws or there would be total chaos.

When then asked, "While I understand what you are saying, others I've asked this same question would disagree with you and say 'They should run the light.' Would you be right, and they are wrong?" "I think they're wrong. They *shouldn't break the law but that is my opinion*. I can't say what somebody else should do." When then asked, "So are you still right and they are wrong or are you equally right?" The Stage 4 subjective response would be, "*We are equally right*," and it might be added, consistent with subjective reasoning, "*I can't say what someone else should do*."

If the person is *relativistic*, they would respond to the last question by saying directly, "It is really arbitrary what a person should do." Or "Words like good, bad, moral and immoral really have no meaning. *You do something because you either want to or do not want to do something*."

Post-conventional Moral Reasoning

And, lastly, the Post-conventional person would indicate having taken into consideration human rights. For example, "They should stop, look both ways, and make sure no one is coming and then run the light?" When asked for their meaning or reasoning of this last statement, they would say or indicate that,

The law is for protecting human life, or our right to our life or existence would pertain to any human life. *Once that is taken care of by stopping and checking that no one is coming from the other direction and having a green light, then the reason for the law or its purpose, or the spirit of the law or the principle underlying the law to protect life would then be to run the red light to save his life.*

If probed and asked additionally, "Others disagree with what you said and think that they should not break the law and they should stop. Are you right and they are wrong, or are you equally right." Their response would be: "*They would be wrong*, because they are not understanding the basis for our having laws which is to protect human life."

Notes to the Practitioner: Clinically Identifying Moral Subjectivism or Relativism

In order to clinically identify moral subjectivism or relativism when using one of the three above moral dilemmas, it is important to determine first, whether or not the person indicates some degree of moral subjectivity in their responses. To determine moral subjectivity, the practitioner would identify whether or not the individual actually has a moral opinion; the moral relativist would have no moral opinion. If moral subjectivity or having a personal opinion is determined, then moral relativism can be ruled out.

Clinically Determining Placement of Subjectivism or Relativism

When, there are indicators of potential transitioning between moral Stage 3 and 4, between moral Stages 4 and 5 or 5 and 6, it is salient to determine the individual's placement in the moral developmental sequence. This is important for the purpose of being able to respond appropriately to couples' predominant moral stage and their potential for transitioning to the next and more adequate stage of moral reasoning (Criterion 4, Chapter 1, p. 2). Understanding which stage(s) is comprehended as well as being questioned/rejected will suggest the predominant stage of moral reasoning. For example, if the practitioner identifies the individual is at moral Stage 3 with potential of transitioning to moral Stage 4, then responding through Socratic questioning the individual *one stage above their own*, which would be the moral reasoning of Stage 4 would then be appropriate.

As another example, during late adolescence/or early adulthood, a young couple, one or both of which are, experiencing identity questioning and confusion, rebelling against societal norms, comprehend Stage 3 and are confused about and questioning, even rejecting the actual value of rules or laws would suggest the possibility of a potential transition between Stages 3 and 4. On the other hand, a couple in which one or both indicate an awareness of the ubiquity of moral subjectivity, perhaps also experiencing identity questioning and confusion in their attempt to find resolution because they are not yet able to construct philosophical reasoning or principles that ought to be an underlying basis of laws, would be suggestive of a potential transition from Stage 4 to 5.

Lastly it is important and therefore being emphasized again, that the individual who is morally subjective, *does have a personal moral viewpoint.* However, because Stage 3 and Stage 4 moral subjectivists consider morality to be personal or subjective, their moral reasoning is that it is also logical that everyone has the same "right" to have their own subjective moral point of view. It is curious however that it is consistently not realized in the slavery dilemma that the enslaved person is denied their human rights. Consistent with this logic, as earlier said, while they do think their moral judgment(s) is correct/right, they will not say that another's moral point of view is necessarily wrong, even if they, personally, believe it to be. Whilst other(s) moral beliefs diametrically opposed to their own, rather than considering it wrong, they believe, and therefore would say in response to the above slavery, Heinz, or chicken bone dilemmas, that both theirs and the diametrically opposing moral judgment of others' are equally right. The moral subjectivist person's moral reasoning then, is, again independent of the conditions, consequences, or the nature of any given objective reality; it is based solely on what one personally or subjectively believes to be true in the given circumstances.

It is critically important that the couple, for their own development, to come to the recognition and identification, for themselves, of the mistaken reasoning of morally subjective or relativistic thinking. This awareness is necessary although not always sufficient to create a reflective form of questioning of one's own moral reasoning along with the resultant cognitive-conflict or disequilibrium necessary for moral growth; the practitioner, as noted, having this awareness can *encourage* this process through Socratic questioning, and the use of the Conceptual Template, and most importantly, *without telling* the couple what or how they should think.

It is further noteworthy for the practitioner to be cognizant that the moral relativist have been aware of subjectivity over an extended period of time, and while perhaps having addressed this issue numerous times, is nevertheless unable to resolve it, and therefore, "resolves" it by "evolving" their awareness of the ubiquitous phenomenon of moral subjectivism into a philosophically "sophisticated" relativistic *stance* or a somewhat enigmatic psychological posture held as an ultimate truth. Because they have constructed a rationale justifying both their metaphysical and meta-ethical position, relativists can be "stabilized," or take a stance that is dogmatically, and subjectively considered to be true, that is, without question, or, is absolutistic.

Given that the individuals/couples will be more or less developed in their moral reasoning/judgment, some will be structurally stabilized, others in some form of disequilibrium, such as between stages, or in transition, and most will to some degree be subjective and even fewer will be entrenched in "morally" relativistic thinking. There can also be those couples that have developed to Post-conventional reasoning, however this occurrence is rare, approximately 15%. Whether more or less developed, individually or as a couple, stabilized or in transition between Stage 3 and 4 (Colby, 1978, Ries, 1979). or between Stages 4 and 5, and even between Stages 5 and 6, all require for this approach to result in the facilitation of both cognitive and cognitive-moral development, an *understanding of the mistaken reasoning of moral subjectivism or relativism.*

It is also possible that the mistaken reasoning of relativism, albeit potentially a transition to Post-conventional Stage 5 moral reasoning/judgment can alternatively, because of confusion and perhaps frustration, result in re-stabilization in either Conventional Stage 3 or 4 or more likely a mixture of the two. Or as stated, the relativistic position can be maintained in a "stabilized" rigid adherence to a meta-ethical and metaphysical stance or assertion taking the position that there is no objective way for determining what is morally right or wrong, and therefore one can do whatever they want. This relativistic unforgiving position, for obvious reasons can be severely problematic in couples' relationships and therefore, again it is being emphasized. On the other hand, and on a more positive note, the practitioner who is aware that, moral relativism can also be a potential transition to Post-conventional Stage 5 moral reasoning, also has the opportunity to specifically apply the Conceptual Template to resolve this form of mistaken or erroneous reasoning, resulting in the facilitation of Principled Stage 5 moral judgment/reasoning.

It is critically important for both practitioner and the couple being counseled to understand the inadequacy of the constructs of both moral subjectivism and/or relativism. Both of these constructs, whether it is subjectivism or the more extreme form of relativism, is suggesting in essence, "who is to say what is moral?" Their erroneous answer to this question: is no one person, it is up to each individual even if they have differing ideas of what is just, including and not withstanding even polar opposite ideas. Or the more extreme form of this phenomenon can be taken, suggesting in essence, that there is no such thing as morality or no objective method for determining, that which is fair or just. The contradictory nature of this phenomenon or more precisely, the awareness of its being contradictory, along with the understanding and use of the Conceptual Template process can result in moral development to Post-conventional moral judgment/reasoning rather than re-stabilizing in Conventional moral reasoning

(Stages 3 and/or 4) or resolving this confusion by philosophical relativism. To say this directly, *the inherent mistaken reasoning of moral subjectivism and it more extreme extrapolation, moral relativism is the fundamental basis or universal underpinnings of moral conflict and injustice.* This is true for humanity and therefore couples.

Reasonable and rational people or couples can come to agreement with regard to resolving moral conflicts or concerns. Defining and understanding the interrelationship of those concepts the mind *naturally* uses in order to understand experience can mitigate and resolve moral conflict. The Conceptual Template is representative of this cognitive and cognitive-moral developmental process. Being consciously aware or mindful of the Conceptual Template provides the conceptual "tools" for being able to universally agree as to that which exists or the nature of things, as does the scientific method. It also provides through objective reasoning as represented in the Conceptual Template, a natural means to not only make life more intelligible, but to also use as a guide in resolving conflicts of claims in what can objectively be agreed upon by rational and reasonable people as universally, fair or just.

Discovering the Conceptual Template process and then being able, through the conscious awareness or mindfulness of these naturally occurring and essential ideas and their interrelationships improves objectivity in our reasoning both in the non-moral and moral realm of human experiences. Objectivity can improve mindfulness of our own subjectivity and that of others. It can also enhance our awareness of the proclivity of subjectivity within ourselves as well as in that of others, resulting in having greater *empathy*. And, most importantly, objective reasoning is necessary for our survival, improving our lives, and interactions with others, the latter of which is the subject matter of this book, that is, the development of moral reasoning improving couples relationship.

Our human nature is one of having an innate rational ability, capable of developing from our naturally occurring subjective experiences to our potential use of greater objectivity in our reasoning in order to improve our understanding of the reality experienced. Our faculty of reason is not only our means of survival and continued existence, but also our means to improving our lives. Our actions in the non-moral realm of experience are not based upon arbitrary means; we would not have continued to exist or survive without the realization of the importance and necessity of objective reasoning. What has not been so evident, is that, for one, what has been implicitly brought to light with the insight that can be gleaned from Kohlberg's longitudinal research describing the naturally occurring invariant sequence of stages within the framework of cognitive and cognitive-moral development, is, the reason that this cognitive awareness used in survival, or improving life, is unlikely to be generalized to moral concerns. One reason, according to Kohlberg is the occurrence of what has been termed the "Naturalist fallacy" namely, confusing that which is, with what ought to be. Because it is recognized in human experience that morality is in fact ubiquitously interpreted subjectively, whether the perception is based upon differing beliefs of individuals, cultures, or religions, it is therefore "logical," actually the mistaken reasoning, to conclude, that it is the way it ought to be. Everybody thinks differently about morality, namely subjectively, therefore who can say what is in reality moral; it is personal. No one wants to be told or preached to by others with regard to what is moral and therefore no one accordingly should judge what is right or wrong for anyone else. Another reason, at least in part, for this mistaken thinking, is that, individuals develop through an invariant sequence of moral stages as described by Kohlberg from being subjective to progressing to universality, or being more objective, and furthermore moral development is a lengthy process from childhood through adulthood.

Although Kohlberg was not prescriptive, but rather descriptive of moral stage development, implicitly, if not explicitly, the more developed stages are objectively more adequate in resolving moral conflict. Stage 6, the most developed or most adequate Post-conventional stage, is explicitly described by Kohlberg as having the capability of rational thought such that it culminates in an orientation which has the capability of resolving moral conflict in a just manner that is, in a manner which is reversible and universalizable. No other stage has that capability; it is the most developed stage of moral reasoning based upon rationality and objectivity. Kohlberg described moral development, in cognitive-moral developmental terms, in that when development from one stage to the next more adequate stage occurs, it is because the disequilibrium or conflict within a stage, finds a way to resolve the cognitive discrepancy or contradiction, not only in terms of logic, rationality, and objective reasoning itself, but objectively in our experiences of the reality in which we live.

The question that remained, however, was not only how to facilitate moral development in general, but more specifically to the most adequate stage(s) of moral reasoning. The answer to this question of how to facilitate moral development is through conceptualizing and integrating essential philosophical concepts for making life more intelligible. This system of reasoning discovered by the individual or couple can create a conscious awareness or mindfulness for understanding and resolving cognitive discrepancies, contradiction, or mistaken reasoning, and in this instance, the mistaken reasoning of the naturalistic fallacy. This therapeutic approach is the subject matter of Chapter 9 and 10.

Organization of the Conceptual Template

Before delineating the Conceptual Template, several comments are relevant regarding the concepts and organization of this framework. The Conceptual Template was constructed based upon earlier research findings. These findings indicated that individuals becoming aware of and then consciously conceptualizing and integrating essential philosophical concepts of rational thought resulted in the facilitation of moral development (Ries, 1979, 1981, 1992/2006). Those individuals who developed to Post-conventional moral judgment/reasoning also resolved the inherent confusion and mistaken reasoning of subjectivism/relativism.

The Conceptual Template utilizes essential philosophical concepts or ideas that were found to be a natural occurrence during a potential transitioning period from Conventional to Post-conventional moral reasoning (Ries, 1979). These concepts appeared to be used in order to understand that which was being experienced, to resolve confusion, as well as to construct meaning (Ries, 1979). The Conceptual Template is a construct of these naturally occurring concepts, which are discovered during couple counseling through Socratic questioning, the purpose of which is to bring these essential concepts to the foreground of consciousness-awareness or mindfulness. When greater clarity of the interrelation of these ideas is required a more Didactic method is used. By becoming mindful or consciously aware of the interrelationship of these essential ideas, the Conceptual Template process can then be used in a more rationally consistent non-contradictory manner, or more objectively. When these concepts were objectively applied through the use of the Conceptual Template, specifically to moral judgment/reasoning, results of a double-blind study found a significant facilitative effect in moral development (Ries, 1981, 1992/2006). This process was also found, in particular and more significantly, to stimulate the ability to construct Principled Stage 5 moral reasoning (Ries, 1981, 1992/2006).

The significance or importance of facilitating Stage 5 moral judgment/reasoning is that Principled Stage 5 moral reasoning is no longer rule-oriented (Stage 4), which can be limiting in scope or inadequate due to its specificity or greater probability for subjectivity. A Principled Stage 5 moral orientation bases decisions on understanding the reasoning of the underlying principles, which are the basis for individual's human rights. This leads to greater adequacy in resolving conflict in a manner that objectively identifies the principles underlying rules, and their interrelation with individuals' human rights. And, within the context of this book, facilitating moral development through the use of the Conceptual Template process resulted in improving couple interaction and intimacy. Progressing in moral development paralleled or resulted in couples having a greater awareness and adequacy in their judgments of how they should treat one another in a manner that is more equitable or just. It is suggested that another reason that couples treat one another more equitably is that integrating these essential concepts results in viewing their significant other not in terms of some social role expectation, but rather seeing their partner through eyes of a universal conceptualization, that is, of being a person.

Foundation of the Conceptual Template

The basis for the construction of the Conceptual Template occurred somewhat serendipitously while overhearing Kohlberg with colleagues in a discussion involving a description of several individuals in Kohlberg's longitudinal research who appeared to be in transition from Conventional Stage 4 to Post-conventional Stag 5 moral reasoning. These individuals, according to Kohlberg and his colleagues appeared to also be experiencing both identity and moral confusion/questioning, the latter of which was in the form of relativism. Their discussion of these psychological events, namely the possible involvement of identity and moral confusion in transitioning to Post-conventional moral reasoning, and even explaining what appeared to be an enigmatic "regression" in moral judgment during this period, were of interest and importance; however, what I heard, or what stood out to me, was, that certain, and very specific ideas appeared to consistently be of concern to these individuals in potential transition when questioning and being confused about their identity and morality. After the meeting, I asked Kohlberg if these ideas – that appeared to me to be consistently reflected upon or questioned during this naturally occurring potential period of moral development – could provide a means for facilitating Post-conventional moral judgment? If these ideas were integrated and their meaning and interrelationship understood, they resolved the mistaken reasoning leading to the manifestation of relativism, subjectivism, or the confusion with respect to their identity. After all, it was what seemed to be necessary and part of the natural struggle for these individuals in a potential transition to Post-conventional Stage 5 moral reasoning. This query led to preliminary research (Ries, 1979).

The preliminary research that followed our discussion focused on the psychological phenomenon of moral relativism, as a potential transition from Conventional Stage 4 and Principled Stage 5 moral reasoning, and its interrelationship with identity formation in moral development (Ries 1979). It was found that identity questioning/confusion and moral questioning/confusion were interrelated. More specifically, it was found, as Kohlberg had earlier suggested (personal communication, Turiel, 1972), that the transition from Conventional (Stage 4) to Principled (Stage 5) moral reasoning did involve a period of reflective questioning and confusion – manifested initially in moral relativism and identity confusion occurring contemporaneously. The resolution of this period of disequilibrium, however, was not found to necessarily result or to be a transition to Principled Stage 5 moral reasoning. Rather this period of questioning/confusion was also resolved in the integration of a stage of moral reasoning consonant with self-concept. Stabilization in Conventional moral judgment (Stages 3 and 4) was found to be associated with a self-concept based upon a particular social role. This was congruent with values conceived in social role terms (what a good husband or wife should do) or values of a Conventional social order (laws should be obeyed). Other individuals who maintained relativism in a more integrated form adopted unconventional identities with commensurate "moral values" which differ from conventional culture in its "extreme relativism" (Kohlberg and Gilligan, 1971). Those who developed to principled moral reasoning (Stage 5) had integrated a universal conceptualization of self, namely defining of self in terms of being human rather than in terms of a particular social role. This conceptualization is congruent with conceptualizing and articulating universal principles regarding such issues as right to life, liberty, and respect for human dignity. To progress to Principled or Post-conventional moral reasoning appeared to require a transformation of self from that of a social role identity to that of universal conceptualization of self.

It was also indicated in the findings of the preliminary research that when individuals were in the early phase of identity and moral questioning/confusion they were asking themselves in the particular "Who am I?" or "Who is the real me?" or similar questioning regarding self-concept. At the same time, they were asking, again in the particular "What do I morally value?" or "How do I really know what is morally right or wrong?" During the later phase of questioning/confusion, the form of reflection was more universal in orientation; for example asking "What does it mean to be human?" or "What is the moral nature of human beings?" In addition, this latter type of inquiry involved an even more general philosophical questioning in what could also be interpreted as seeking an understanding of life's meaning or resolving some form of existential confusion/anxiety, asking various but similar types of questions in an attempt to resolve their confusion or concerns. The same concepts that stood out in Kohlberg's discussion with his colleagues regarding his subjects in what appeared to be a potential transition were again found to be especially salient to the individuals in the preliminary research when questioning and reflecting upon specific ideas or concepts in their attempt to resolve their disequilibrium. These questions and similar ones, when understood and integrated, were found in the preliminary study to result in a universal identity with corresponding universal principles. The type of questions expressed in various ways but consistently were:

Who am I?
What is the meaning of my existence?
Who is the real me?
What is truth?
How do I know what is real?
How do I know anything?
How do I know that everything is not just a dream?
How do I know if what I perceive is true?
How do I know that I know?
How do I know what is really worthwhile, or of value?
What does it mean to be human?
What is good?
What is evil?
How do I know what is good or evil?
What is my true nature?
What is moral?
Is what I value merely what I believe, or a matter of opinion?
Is morality merely a matter of opinion or belief (subjective)?
What is reality?
Is there any way to understand or to know what is moral?
How do I understand anything for sure?
Is there some (objective) way to answer these questions in order to understand what I am living?

Asking these types of questions, in what appeared to be an attempt to resolve their identity and moral confusion, the individuals in the preliminary study also consistently focused on very specific and essential philosophical ideas, again as did Kohlberg's subjects. These ideas centered on reality, illusion, truth, knowledge, opinion, belief, subjectivity, objectivity, value, good and evil, morality, and justice. Philosophers such as Socrates, revealed through the writing of Plato, himself, and Aristotle, to mention a few were in particular also concerned with these very specific ideas. They spent much time attempting to define and interrelate these essential concepts. It appeared then that these philosophers and individuals in the preliminary study, as did Kohlberg's subjects in potential transition, focused specifically on the same and essential ideas or concepts. As mentioned in the introduction, that these great thinkers focused on these identical ideas that humans have difficulty understanding may not be coincidental.

What seemed to be the "missing link" that philosophers and these individuals were focused on resolving was a consistent and rational logic or non-contradictory system of reasoning that could be used to objectively construct meaning, that is, a means by which to make life more intelligible. Defining and interrelating the ideas or essential concepts that these great thinkers also focused on and/or thought to be particularly important led to the construction of the Conceptual Template. This system of reasoning could be used to have descriptive knowledge of reality, that is, matters of fact and existence, or what is. It would serve to facilitate a conscious awareness of these ideas and the means by which one could perceive more clearly, logically and rationally, one's own or others thinking/reasoning through verbal communication, whether with regard to the existence of occurrences in reality outside of one's control or the events or interactions of life within one's control. It can also serve to more objectively identify resolutions that are equitable in a particular set of circumstances. Between couples, this system or reasoning could be used to better resolve challenges of differences in opinions, preferences, cultural differences, or conflict regarding individuals as well as their rights and beliefs.

The hypotheses that evolved from this preliminary research then, was that by simulating a natural process or system of reasoning, depicted in, the Conceptual Template, could facilitate what appeared to also occur naturally in moral development in the transition from Conventional (Stage 4) to Principled (Stage 5) moral reasoning/judgment as well as the development of one's identity or self-concept. A double-blind study supported the preliminary research findings that a system of reasoning of conceptualizing and integrating essential philosophical concepts can result in the integration of a stage of moral reasoning consonant with self-concept, as well as both significantly facilitate moral development in general and Post-conventional moral judgment/reasoning in particular (Ries, 1981, 1992/2006).

Summary

The construction of the Conceptual Template process then was based upon what initially and serendipitously appeared to be an innate or natural process in human development during a process of transitioning from Conventional to Post-conventional moral judgment/reasoning. This was first noticed when subjects during this potential transitioning period appeared to consistently focus on very specific concepts in their attempts to resolve their confusion with regard to their identity and morality.

Research findings that the resolution of identity and moral confusions could lead to Post-conventional Principled Stage 5 moral judgment/reasoning through integrating these essential ideas, led to seeking a means by which to replicate or re-create this process through the formulation or the construct of the Conceptual Template.

Chapter 10

Universal Conceptual Template Program

The Conceptual Template reveals a universal system of reasoning dis-covered by the couple through the identification, conceptualization, and integration of specific and essential philosophical concepts. It provides a logical, systematic and non-contradictory approach to improving the nat-ural ability to think more rationally and objectively. It reveals an objective thinking process that can enhance critical thinking skills. And, the Con-ceptual Template can facilitate moral development. In essence the Con-ceptual Template empowers couples or individuals, with a consistent, non-contradictory, and rational means of understanding one another and applying their reasoning ability to problem-solving and decision making in a manner that is equitable. Ultimately this conceptual mindfulness results in improving communication and intimacy in couples' relationships.

The construction of the Conceptual Template began with Aristotle's declaration on the importance of definition and meaning in reasoning and understanding things (1952, p. 525):

> If one were to say the word has an infinite number of meanings, obviously reasoning would be impossible; for not to have one meaning is to have no meaning and if words have no meaning our reasoning with one another, and indeed with ourselves, has been annihilated; for it is impossible to think of anything if we do not think of one thing.

Using classical philosophical definitions, particularly those of Plato and Aristotle, each concept that appeared essential to both Kohlberg's subjects and individuals in the preliminary research who were in potential transi-tion to Post-conventional moral judgment/reasoning, were interrelated into a rational-logical non-contradictory objective framework.

The Conceptual Template evolved with the following being kept in mind.

> There are more things in heaven and earth, Horatio,
> than are dreamt in your philosophy.
> (Shakespeare, 1947)

CONCEPTUAL TEMPLATE

PART ONE - A RATIONAL THINKING PROCESS

STEPS

I. Experience	**REALITY**
II. Interpret	**ACTUALITY**
III. Question	**TRUE CORRECT** P R O O F **FALSE INCORRECT**
IV. Verify	**NOT KNOW** **KNOWLEDGE** **NOT SURE**

PART TWO - APPLICATION OF THE PROCESS

V. Criteria	**VALUES**
and	
Evaluation	**RIGHTS**
VI. Judgment	**MORALITY**
and	
Action	**JUSTICE**

©1995, Human Development Institute

Table 10.1 Universal Conceptual Template

Human consciousness and the faculty of reason enable individuals to be aware of experience. In Step I, with experience as a beginning, it can be asked or reflected upon, "*What is it that we experience?*" The answer to this question is, for operational purposes, **Reality?** It is what comes in through our senses, is integrated, and then conceptualized, which again for operational purposes is our *Actuality or our interpretation of our experience of a reality*, which leads us to Step II. Our experiences of reality may vary, nevertheless, as expressed by great thinkers, such as Socrates/Plato, and Aristotle to mention a few, reality is, in essence, what is, that which exists or the nature of things. *This is not to say what a particular reality is, it is merely saying that reality is, what it is, no matter how it is perceived or interpreted by any person.*

When Step III is reached, we see that **Reality** is the state of things, as they actually exist and therefore it follows that our **Actuality**, *interpretations*, conceptualizations, or constructs of a reality are objectively, either **True** or **False**. In other words, our interpretation or what we think, or our **Actuality**, actually corresponds to reality or it does not. It is suggested that this is a self-evident truth. Again as Aristotle makes us aware, stating in more words or less, "something cannot both be and not be at the same time."

It is a natural human tendency, to think that what we initially think, or that our own interpretation or **Actuality** is true. This human response is necessary so we can take immediate action when survival is at a crucial moment; Plato in the *Allegory of the Cave*, as earlier mentioned, poignantly illustrated this initial and reactive reasoning. Conflict may be experienced when reacting to an initial **Actuality**. It is a natural occurrence to question or to interpret reality in an attempt to understand what is or what it is that we are experiencing. We are capable of questioning our own initial **Actuality** as well, which is what we think is, or interpret what is occurring/happening; this begins the process of determining decisive action versus initial reaction. By consciously questioning our initial Actuality or reasoning, we are better equipped to determine what is **True** in **Reality**. In a composite **Actuality** we can then decide on our actions versus an initial reaction. Human interactions or relationships may experience less conflict and greater ability to resolve complex dilemmas in a fair or just manner by heightening awareness that our initial **Actuality** may be true or false and therefore initial reactions may be questioned and reconstructed as well. In terms of evolution this may have been the natural progression for human survival. By questioning our initial **Actuality** or **Actualities**, this provided the means by which humanity has refined their critical thinking and problem-solving ability.

In our everyday experiences, in order to more objectively identify reality, it is necessary to be mindful of this phenomenon. It is beneficial to question and analyze our initial interpretations/conceptualization(s) and to examine what may be the consequential effects. To begin to determine if an actuality is **True** would be to determine if it, in fact, consistently corresponds to reality. To begin to determine if an actuality were **False** would be to determine if, in fact, it consistently is non-correspondent to reality. It is at this juncture that we may begin to consider that it can be beneficial to our thinking to be more objective and rational about our own and partner's thinking. For example, you can think that your spouse or partner means one thing in a verbal interaction, but by questioning the dialogue and meaning of each individual's **Actuality** we can begin to be more objective. "What is the truth of their intentions and point of view in contrast to our perception, interpretation, or conceptualization of their motive, meaning or expression?" At this point in our cognitive process, we are determining if our Actuality is True in Reality; we want to be correctly informed, our thinking or our *Actuality* will vary based on the information we have, which can lead to unnecessary conflict. Our goal is to better understand one another and the Reality, supporting the necessary communication and understanding to encourage a healthy and intimate relationship.

Case Example

George's wife, Georgette typically finishes work at 5pm and arrives at home approximately 5:50 pm after grocery shopping. Thinking that Georgette will be home at 5:50pm, George begins preparing her a special Valentines dinner accordingly. Georgette worked an extra 30 minutes due to a meeting that she forgot and hasn't mentioned to George; she arrives at 6:30pm. When she arrives home, George is sullen and upset. Dinner is cold. He was very excited to make dinner for Georgette and estimated, she would be home around 5:50pm. George wonders why his wife is late and has worried if something had happened to her. When Georgette arrives home safely, his worry becomes frustrated agitation.

Simple misunderstandings can happen, for example, when we do not have all the same information. George did not know that Georgette would have a meeting and Georgette didn't know he was preparing dinner as he frequently relied on her for dinner preparation. George had wanted to surprise Georgette so he had not told her he was preparing dinner or not to go shopping, instead he attempted to calculate her arrival including her regular shopping time. Georgette had forgotten that she would be having a meeting and did not inform George she would be late. Due to this missing information George was upset over his attempt at surprising his wife and Georgette was confused as to why he was upset.

This confusion and conflict was resolved when they have a conversation about their perceived actualities in a manner that was both rational and objective unraveling the events of the day and their non-communications with each other. Estimating the time Georgette will finish work on a particular day is a simplified example that each *Actuality* of reality is either actually true or false. Each individual's *Actuality* may be objective or subjective in his or her reasoning.

To be *Objective* means the state or quality of being outside of a subject's or individual's biases, interpretations, feelings and imaginings or impressions. To be *Subjective* means that state or quality of being is based on or influenced by feelings, tastes, preferences or opinions. Subjectivities can be true for one person but not necessarily for another person. Sheila likes strawberry ice cream but Leila does not. Our *Actuality* can also be referred to as our perception, interpretation or conceptualization of reality. Our

Perception or Conceptualization of Reality compiles the ability to see, hear, or become aware of something through the senses. It cannot objectively be both correct and incorrect at the same time.

As Aristotle (1952, p. 515) said, "everything must be either affirmed or denied, … a thing cannot at the same time be and not be." Thus, the question to be asked is, "How does one objectively have *Knowledge* of whether what they think, their *Actuality* is in fact true?" (subjectivity/perception). Couples or individuals can realize, be consciously aware, or mindful while going through this process, that their interpretation, *Actuality*, may or may not be true, that we do not automatically or necessarily *Know* whether what we think or our *Actuality* is in fact, true.

Step IV, *Knowledge*, is yet another step in the process of understanding a reality, one which is subsequent to our thinking that our interpretation of a reality is either true or false. To know requires objective proof. Understanding a reality or having knowledge of a reality requires being able to objectively prove an actual correspondence between what one thinks to be true, and reality.

If an Actuality of Reality cannot be objectively proven, this Actuality may be a subjective opinion or belief, which may be the truth for a particular individual or group of similarly reasoning individuals. *Knowledge* by operational definition for this book constitutes the proven correspondence between a thought and reality. While opinion or belief can be either true or false; it is subject to doubt until proven true.

The paradigm up to this point is concerned with understanding the concepts and their interrelationships necessary in comprehending reality. It is objective in that it is concerned with facts excluding desires or wishes. It is objective because the means by which knowledge is acquired is not arbitrary, but is constructed by the rationality of the meaning and interrelationships of those concepts used by humans to understand reality. Further, it is objective in that it proves itself in reality to be correct; it is verifiable.

Up to this point of the paradigm, the scientific community would in general agree that when we are dealing with reality, that is, matters of fact, the nature of things, or real existence, that this approach, although schematic, is one, which can lead objectively to knowledge, even about itself, as does the scientific method. While equipping the human mind of being better able to determine what is Truth and what we Know, the second part of the Conceptual Template encourages the potential of the human mind to determine and prioritize what is of value and what is fair and just. It is at this juncture that the concept of value and evaluation, Step V, or that, which is important or worthwhile to us, is of concern or relevance.

Case Example

Jim and Jolie have a four-year-old son. Jolie is a fashion magazine editor and the breadwinner in the family. She works all hours of the day setting deadlines for prints of the staff writers and freelance writers, supervising staff and reading, writing, researching and proofreading features and articles. Jim is a freelance writer for a journal company who operates in his home office and raises their son Jon.

Jon has a performance for his preschool where the children dress as the previous American presidents and are to give a brief summary or repeat a phrase of that president. Jolie is unable to attend the performance due to an article deadline. Jim and Jolie have their first discussion of the amount of hours she puts in at work since having Jon.

JOLIE: Jon "is getting older now and attending preschool and goes to kindergarten soon, I'm concerned about the amount of hours you're working. He will be needing us both more," says Jim.

"I know Jim, I really wanted to be there for his performance," said Jolie

"I'm wondering if there's anything you can work out with your company management. You've been putting off hiring another assistant editor. It would be really nice if you could have more help at work," Jim suggests.

Jolie considers this for a moment. "Oh Jim, I'm just so busy." She sighs, "It would be wonderful to have the extra help. I've really wanted to try to incorporate a more structured routine for our staff but you know the deadlines we've been dealing with."

"Well," says Jim. "Please remember Jon is getting older every day. It's up to you to find an assistant. The company has already approved the request. I know you love Jon and I think we both want for him to remember both of us being involved in his life. He's old enough to remember what we do and he's absorbing everything like a sponge."

"I do Jim, I promise I'll make some time after this next deadline."

A few weeks have passed and Jim inquires if Jolie has spoken with any potential hires.

"Jolie," asks Jim. "Have you spoken with any potential hires? How's the assistant search going?"

Jolie is quiet for a moment before answering. "I haven't scheduled any interviews just yet."

Jim take a deep breath; this a recurring conversation.

"Jolie, I know you have a lot on your plate but the only way I can see for you to have more time is to take the time to hire more staff."

"I know," expressed Jolie, "I just don't know where I'm going to find the time to even interview anyone."

"Jolie, What's more important, being able to get a better work environment for yourself and your co-workers, being able to spend more time with your family, or avoiding asking for help? Maybe someone else can assist you with selecting interview prospects and even some of the interviews if you ask, but you need to put aside some time to consider that or put aside time to do it yourself."

"You're right Jim, it's easier to supervise the staff and hassle writers to meet their deadlines than it is for me to interview prospects, but I think Wanda may be willing to help and I trust her judgment in selecting and interviewing prospects. Thanks Jim, I will make time to speak with her on this matter. I'll email her now to schedule a small meeting before our staff briefing tomorrow."

"That's great! Two heads are better than one."

"They are. I need to remember missing Jon's performance. Being a part of raising our son is very important and I'm sure everyone at work wants to spend more time with his or her families as well. If we can arrange to have one or two more staff we'll complete the assignments for each deadline with a better pace."

In this example, the couple shared resources to find a resolution and put it into place. Jolie may have been too overwhelmed by all that she had on her plate to put into perspective that she needed to prioritize hiring more staff. Jim really assisted Jolie in taking the time to put into perspective what was happening and what was needed to resolve the issue. By communicating this couple was able to prioritize a resolution and Jolie was able to conceptualize the effects and was ready to act on it. Relationships are an integral part of sharing resources and finding resolutions to problems as well as conflicts. Time and thought are necessary in analyzing situations and establishing resolutions.

The second part of the Conceptual Template takes into account the concept of *Values* or that, which is important or worthwhile and distinguishes between subjectively and objectively derived *Values*. Subjectively derived values are personal and are important to an individual or group of individuals of similar reasoning. Subjectively derived values may vary from individual to individual or group of similar reasoning individuals as they are based on or influenced by feelings, tastes, preferences or opinions, which also vary from individual to individual or similar group of individuals.

Objectively derived values are the same for all people. These values are directly derived from *Reality* with regard to all human physical and metaphysical needs independent of subjective emotion or desire or any particular interpretation of a reality. Needs refer here to that which is inherent in our nature and is universal for human existence, one's quality of life, well-being or happiness, not to that which is acquired and specific to the individual or a particular group of individuals. Objective values are not particular to the individual.

Since objective values are based upon what is of value to humans in reality, they cannot be merely any value important to only some people in particular circumstances of a reality. To be objectively of value, even to a lesser or higher degree it must be of value to all rational people, aware of it or not, in any reality. Anything different would be of subjective value or dependent on a person's particular life circumstances or the reality in which they live at any given time or to which they were, by chance, born. Therefore, it is not a particular reality in which we are born that determines what is important or an objectively derived value, even if appearing so, but rather that which is important in any reality, to any one of us, no matter what the conditions are, in any particular reality to which we are born that is objectively of value to humans in reality. And, it is therefore that which is of value to all rational people, even if not aware of it, that are the basis of our RIGHTS as individuals, which is integral to Step V. The last scenario not only involved both subjectively and objectively derived values, and although perhaps not so apparent, which is usually the case, entailed rights as well.

Since it is the reality for all of us that is being referred to, not a particular reality or circumstances to some, no one has any different relationship to it in terms of being objectively of value. We all have the same relationship to it, or to the nature of reality. We can only survive, exist, sustain our existence and well-being or even be happy by acting or living, at least for the most part, in accordance with reality. And, therefore, it rationally and objectively follows that if it is the reality of that which is being referred to that which is the same for all of us, independent of chance, then, reason and rationality would subscribe to the proposition that we are equally entitled to what is of value to all of us; no rational person would want this to be dictated by chance alone, or the conditions to which we are born. This then is the basis of a human right or more precisely rights. It also follows then, that objectively derived values are what all people are entitled to by virtue of their existence. It is, by definition our RIGHT. As Thomas Paine expressed:

> It is impossible to discover any
> origin of rights otherwise than in the
> origin of man; it consequently follows
> that right appertain to man in right of
> his existence.
>   (Quoted from a Celestial
>   Seasonings tea box)

While we are entitled or have a right to that which is objectively of value in reality to all people, this does not mean we can have or do whatever we want willy-nilly. Human subjectivity of what one might believe they are entitled, can and has led to conflict, with lesser or greater consequences in interactions of people in general and couples in particular. For us to survive and to have a good life we have created a construct; it is, morality, Step VI. Morality can be defined in part as a "code of values that guide our choices and actions..." (Rand, 1986) in situations of conflicting interest, the most important of which are, our, or all of our, rights. And, it is JUSTICE, Step VI, that can determine what any rational human being or person would consider in a situation involving conflicting interests or our rights to be equitable. Any one of us, that is, given that we could be born into any circumstances by chance, and not knowing what position in a conflict of interests we could be in, including the least advantaged position, even if we might subjectively disagree, could not rationally disagree that we could determine, much of the time, a resolution that would be fair or just for all or any of us were we to make our decision as well as accept that choice for ourself not knowing which position we could be in. This was referenced earlier in the use of the principles of reversibility and universalizability as illustrated in Moral Musical Chairs that can serve this purpose.

Summary

The distinction between objectively derived needs (based upon reality) and subjectively derived wants (based upon individuals actuality alone) allows us to state a self-evident truth as a first principle, which is: we *ought* to desire that which is in reality good for us. By using the first principle or prescriptive truth (ought) and adding to it a descriptive truth of reality (in this instance descriptive truth regarding the objective nature of human beings and their needs), we can correctly reach a conclusion that is a further descriptive truth; or knowledge of what is good for us in reality; we *ought* to desire that which is good or beneficial to us (Adler, 1985), namely, that which is reversible and universalizable. Since all objectively derived values, needs or that which is good for us is not equally good; we can develop a hierarchy of what is of greater or lesser value in reality. Those higher on the scale, namely, those things that are required to sustain our existence, or those that have no limit in value such as liberty or knowledge, would supersede values that are only of limited value. Nevertheless, all are natural needs and are, therefore, the basis of our natural rights.

In order for couples to be more objective about their relationship in general and what is of more or less value in particular situations of having serious conflicting interests or rights, they can use the Conceptual Template and the moral principle earlier discussed with the criteria of reversibility and universability as a guide to determine what any or all rational people could agree to were they not to know which position in which they could be, particularly the least advantaged position. This would provide couples with the means by which they could determine what is actually fair or just. Couples can be conscious or mindful then of *how they treat one another which is the essence of moral reasoning*, and also have a rational and objective means in order to best resolve issues of conflict when they occur in their relationship using the organization of the essential ideas of the Conceptual Template as a guide.

The purpose of the Conceptual Template is to learn to be conscious or mindful of how we are reasoning so that we can use this knowledge to not only understand and respond appropriately to our life experiences in general, but in this context, as a guide for resolving human conflict specifically in our relationship with our spouse or significant other. Further, it is the aim of the Conceptual Template to facilitate cognitive development; particularly cognitive-moral development so that conflict can be prevented, and when not, can be resolved equitably or in a just manner. This ultimately results in improved communication, understanding of one another, and intimacy.

Chapter 11

A Conceptual Template for Facilitating Critical Thinking and Ethical Reasoning

Practitioners' Instruction Manual

Purpose of Practitioners' Instructional Manual

- To provide a logical and systematic instructional approach to facilitating couples' (individuals) natural ability to think more objectively and rationally.
- To reveal a natural thinking process through the identification, conceptualization, and integration of specific and essential philosophical concepts.
- To teach and demonstrate how an objective thinking process can enhance critical thinking skills, as well as work in conjunction with recognized styles of learning.
- To empower couples' (individuals) with a consistent and rational means of understanding and applying their reasoning ability to problem solving and decision making, as well as being responsible citizens in a democratically evolving society and world.

The Universal Conceptual Template Program

Overview

The Conceptual Template Program is derived from scientific research conducted at Harvard, which analyzed how individuals naturally use certain philosophical concepts in their reasoning.

From this research it was hypothesized and subsequently validated that a program which objectively intervened in this natural reasoning process could effectively:

a) Facilitate critical thinking
b) Stimulate ethical development
d) Provide a guide for rationally approaching ethical concerns, such that all parties can construct, or agree upon, an objectively derived standard of ethical conduct

Aim

- To teach couples how to identify and understand, through their own thinking, the meaning and interrelationship of specific philosophical concepts which naturally form a conceptual template for rational and objective reasoning or critical thinking.
- To teach couples how to use this Conceptual Template to enhance their Critical Thinking Skills.
- To teach couples how to apply this model for critical thinking to a myriad of life experiences.
- To assist practitioners in teaching critical thinking skills and stimulating ethical development.

Organization

The Conceptual Template is designed to be used by the practitioner as a facilitating tool for guiding couples in the identification of a natural, rational thinking process.

The Template is made up of essential concepts to be identified and agreed upon by the couples. The concepts are an integral part of the natural reasoning process that people use when they think about anything they experience in life.

The Template (framework) represents a Two-Part, Six-Step approach to understanding these essential concepts, and applying them to the development of creative and critical thinking skills, problem-solving, decision-making, and ethical reasoning/judgment.

The Two-Part, Six-Step Template
Part One: A Rational Thinking Process (Steps I–VI)

The First Four Steps teach couples how to identify a natural, logical, and rational conceptual reasoning process that leads to improving critical thinking skills.

STEP I	EXPERIENCING
STEP II	INTERPRETATION
STEP III	QUESTIONING
STEP IV	VERIFICATION

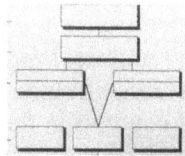

Part Two – Application of a Rational Thinking Process (Steps V, VI)

The Fifth Step identifies the criteria and guidelines necessary for effectively applying one's natural thinking to making important decisions and choices, as well as resolving ethical issues and concern.

STEP V	CRITERIA
	and
	EVALUATION

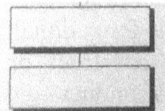

The Sixth Step demonstrates how to determine guidelines for constructing an objectively derived standard for achieving ethical conduct.

STEP VI   JUDGMENT
and
ACTION

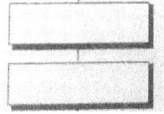

Program Teaching Methods

- **SOCRATIC – Purpose:**

  - To cause cognitive conflict and to support more adequate forms of reasoning
  - To assist couples in operationally defining the meaning of certain essential philosophical concepts, as well as the interrelationships between them.

- **DIDACTIC – Purpose:**

  - To refine the understanding, definition, and interrelationship between these concepts, which are integral to the Conceptual Template.

Suggestions for Effectively Teaching the Template Program

- Establish that reason is the means by which human beings understand reality.
- Establish reason as the authority in determining rational thought and behavior, rather than a particular individual or group.
- Ask couples to discover for themselves how their mind reasons conceptually and rationally.
- Encourage couples to discover for themselves how their mind reasons conceptually and rationally.
- Provide examples that will allow couples to apply the conceptual process (Template).
- Exact wordings of the Socratic Questions are not crucial, however, the identification, understanding, meaning and interrelationship of each concept is essential.
- Establish an operational definition for each concept.
- Review each new concept after an operational definition has been established, and have couples interrelate new concepts with previous ones.
- This facilitates their understanding, as well as reinforces their ability to integrate concepts into their reasoning.

Orienting the Couples

- Operational Definition – Establish the following:

- The importance of defining terms/words – to create clarity and consistency within one's thinking.
- The importance of recognizing the meaning of terms/words – to communicate and understand what each person is expressing.

- Couple Orientation – Establish the following:

  - There is a natural conceptual process for thinking that all people use when they think about what they sense, perceive and experience.
  - Couples will learn how to identify, understand, and apply this process in order to enhance their critical thinking skills, and make ethical decisions.

Teaching Manual Format

The Conceptual Template Teaching Manual provides practitioners with the following step-by-step, interactive format specifically designed to be self-contained unit, or to be integrated into any content area, as well as to work in conjunction with recognized learning styles.

CONTENT FOCUS	UNDERSTANDING GOALS
Each step contains one or more related concepts/ideas, which are to be identified by the couples	The identification of the meaning of the concepts/ideas to be learned and understood by the couples
Socratic Questions Questions or prompts the practitioner uses to elicit the identification and/or meaning of a concept.	**Typical Responses of Individuals** Responses couples give to Socratic questions regarding concepts and their meaning. Practitioner may use couples' responses to engage in discussion in order to determine which concept best applies and why.
Check Questions Rephrasing of the Socratic questions practitioners ask to reconfirm the couples' understanding of the concepts and their specific meaning (operational definition).	**Check Answers** Couples' responses to the check questions after discussing their typical responses to the Socratic questions.

Conceptual Template Program Concepts/Ideas

The following represents a collection of concepts/ideas suggested by couples as important.

A
Actuality
Accommodate
Adaptation
Appreciation
Assimilate
Attitude
Authority
Awareness

B
Bad
Being
Belief
Beneficial

C
Calmness
Categorizing
Character
Choice
Communication
Comparison
Compassion
Conclusion
Confidence
Consistency
Contentment
Correct
Correlation
Courage
Creativity

D
Deception
Development
Differentiate
Discernment
Discrimination
Diversity

E
Effect
Empathy
Empirical
Emotion
Ethics
Evaluate
Experience

F
Fact
Fairness
Faith
Falsity
Fantasy
Fear
Feeling
Forgiveness
Freedom
Fulfillment

G
Goals
God
Good
Growth
Guilt

H
Happiness
Harm
History
Honesty
Honor
Humor hurt
Hypothesis

I
Ignorance
Illusion
Immoral importance
Incorrect
Independence
Individual
Inference
Intuition
Irrational

J
Judgment
Justice

K
Knowledge

P
Passion
Peace perception
Pessimistic
Pleasure

Positive
Possibilities
Potential
Predictable
Principle
Priorities
Process
Proof
Prosperity
Purpose

Q
Question

R
Rational
Rationalization
Reality
Reason
Reflection
Relationship
Relativity
Respect
Right
Rights

S
Satisfaction
Self
Sensitivity
Senses
Standard
Stillness
Subjectivity
Success
Survival
Sympathy

T
Thinking
Thought
Tolerance
True
Truth

V
Value

W
Wisdom
Wit

The Universal Conceptual Template

Part One – A Rational Thinking Process (Steps I–VI)

Teaching the Template

Step I: Experience

Content Focus: Reality	Understanding Goals
• The condition that all human beings experience and are part of is called reality • To survive and improve life we need to understand reality • The meaning of the word reality can be perceived/interpreted differently by different people • Reality exists independent of perceptions or interpretations	• Reality is what we experience and need to understand • We need to understand reality to survive and improve life • People can perceive/interpret different meanings of the word "reality" • Reality exists independent of one's perceptions or interpretations

First: Socratic Questions	Typical Responses of Individuals
• What is it we are experiencing all of the time? • What is it we are sensing all of the time? • What is it we are perceiving all of the time? • What is it we are trying to identify all of the time? • What is it we are always needing and trying to understand?	• Various concepts, such as Life, Nature, Reality • Various concepts • Various concepts • Various concepts • Various concepts

Check Question	Check Answer
What is it we are experiencing, sensing, perceiving, trying to identify and understand all of the time?	Reality is what we experience through our senses and seek to understand.

Second: Socratic Question	Typical Responses of Individuals
• Why is it important to understand reality?	• To survive • To make sense of things • To communicate and relate with others • To improve or make life better • To have a good life – to be happy

Check Question	Check Answer
Why is it important to understand reality?	We need to understand reality to survive, and improve or have a good life

PRACTIONER'S NOTE: The purpose of the third Socratic question on the following page is not to have the couple specifically define the meaning of the word reality, rather it is meant to demonstrate that reality can mean different things to different people, which can lead to confusion.

Third: Socratic Question (Transitional Point)	Typical Responses of Individuals
Since we all have to understand reality in order to survive, and improve or have a good life, what do we mean by the word "reality"?	• Reality is what is tangible or what you can touch • Reality is different for everyone • Reality is truth • Reality is actual fact, or facts • Reality is the way things are, or what is • Reality is how a person perceives it to be • Reality is what a person believes to be true • Reality is an illusion or a dream. (Nihilism)

Check Question	Check Answer
• What does it tell us when people have a different meaning of reality?	• People can have a different idea as to what reality means

Fourth: Socratic Questions (Transitional Point)	TYPICAL RESPONSES OF INDIVIDUALS
• If one does not perceive a reality, does that mean that it does not exist? (Plato's tree in the forest.)	• Yes, or no
• If people have different interpretations of reality, does that mean that there is no reality?	• Yes, no, varied and confused

Practitioner's Note:

• Couples tend to experience cognitive conflict (confusion) in their thinking at this point, which is natural; therefore nothing needs to be done at this time. Confusion allows for new questioning, and potential development.

Check Question	Check Answer
• If people do not perceive a reality, or have different interpretations of reality, does that mean that there is no reality, or that reality does not exist?	• No, it means that people can interpret reality differently

Step II: Interpretation

Content Focus: Actuality	Understanding Goals

• People can interpret reality differently
 	
   • Actuality is introduced to differentiate between what people experience (Reality), and how they actually interpret their experience of reality (Actuality)
 	
   • Optional – review the Third and fourth Socratic Question in Step I, namely that reality can mean different things to different people, and that people can have different interpretations of reality
 	
• One person cannot interpret the same reality differently from another; and contradict each other; and both be correct
 	
• Operationally define the meaning of the word 'reality'
	• People can interpret the same reality in different ways
	
	• When using an objective thinking process, contradictory interpretations of the same reality are either correct or incorrect, but both cannot be correct
	
	• Reality is that which exists; reality is the nature of things; reality is what is, no matter how we perceive or interpret it

First: Socratic Question	Typical Couple Response
• Can there be a difference between what a reality is and the way we interpret it to be?	• Yes; reality can be interpreted differently by different people
Check Question	**Check Answer**
• Can people interpret reality differently?	• People can have different interpretations of reality

Practitioner's Note:

- Introduce the ideas of subjectivity and objectivity.
- Subjectivity is basing what one holds to be true or false on one's feelings or interpretations alone, rather than upon the attributes of the object itself or the reality being considered.
- Objectivity is focusing upon the attributes or characteristics of the object itself or the reality being considered; it excludes desires in considering the truth.
- Using examples, establish the meaning and differences between objective and subjective thinking.
- By being aware of one's own and other's subjectivity an individual can be more objective in his/her own thinking.

Second: Socratic Question	Typical Responses of Individuals
• If one interprets reality one way and someone else's interpretation contradicts it, can they both be correct?	• They can both be right • One is right and one is wrong • Neither one is right

Check Question	Check Answer
• Can people interpret the same reality differently and both be correct?	• Objectively, contradictory interpretations of the same reality are either correct or incorrect, but both cannot be correct

Practitioner's note:

• If couples respond with "both can be right," then introduce examples regarding objective and subjective thinking, then point out that this only applies in the case of subjective interpretations, likes or dislikes, preferences, or tastes; however, this does not change the objective nature of the reality being perceived.

Third: Socratic Question	Typical Responses of Individuals
• Based upon the ideas we have discussed so far, what do we mean by the word reality?	• Life • What is • The way things are • What is happening

Check Questions	Check Answer
• How would you define the word reality?	• Reality is that which exists or the nature of things

Practitioner's note:

• Review the meaning of operational definitions.
• Review the idea of actuality (one's interpretation of reality).
• Using examples, such as, "Is it a pen or a pencil?" demonstrate the difference between one's experience of reality (objective), as a condition, and actuality (subjective), as one's interpretation of the reality being experienced.

Step III: Questioning

Content Focus: True, False, Correct or Incorrect	Understanding Goals
• In order to be more objective in our thinking about reality it is important to question whether our interpretation (actuality) is true or false, correct or incorrect, in reality • People can think that what they think is true, even if it is not • The couples will learn how to determine the meaning of truth (what is true) in relation to reality • The couples will learn how to determine the meaning of falsity (what is false) in relation to reality • Objectively determining whether one's thinking/ideas are true or false can create order and understanding in one's thinking, and can lead to correctly identifying reality	• In order to be objective in one's thinking, individuals must realize that their interpretation (actuality) of a reality must be either true or false • A person's thoughts or ideas may or may not be true • True or truth is a thought or statement which corresponds to reality • Falsity is a thought or statement which contradicts reality • Individuals can create order and understanding in their thinking/ ideas by objectively determining what is true or false in reality, which can lead to enhancing survival, improving life and communicating more clearly

Practitioner's note:

• Step II leads to Step III: Once we experience reality, and begin to interpret it (actuality), the next step (III) is to question whether our interpretation (actuality) of reality is true or false, unless it is subjective or self-evident.

First: Socratic Question	Typical Responses of Individuals
• In order to be more objective in our thinking about reality we must question and recognize that any interpretation of reality is either _____ or _____?	• Right or wrong • True or false • Correct or incorrect • Real or not real
Check Question	**Check Answer**
• Our interpretation of reality has to be either _____ or _____?	• Our interpretation of reality is either true or false

Practitioner's note:

- To clarify the couples' understandings of this question ask, "Can something be both true and false at the same time"?
- Maintain the idea of this being an objective thinking process with regard to reality, rather than one's personal subjective experiences, tastes, preferences, opinions, likes or dislikes.
- The reasoning is that someone can think that a thought/idea is either true or false; however, someone cannot rationally think that a thought/idea can be both true and false at the same time.

Second: Socratic Question	**Typical Responses of Individuals**
• Are the thoughts or ideas in your mind always true?	• It's true to you • No
Check Question	**Check Answer**
• Because you think something to be true or correct, does that make it true or correct?	• Your thoughts or ideas in your mind are either true or false

Third: Socratic Question	**Typical Responses of Individuals**
• What is the definition of true or truth	• What's real • A synonym for reality • Proof that something is real • Honesty • Your own feelings • What's correct • That which is actual
Check Question	**Check Answer**
• What do we mean by something being true?	• True or truth means that what is thought or said corresponds to reality
Fourth: Socratic Question	**Typical Responses of Individuals**
• What is the definition of false?	• Opposite of truth • Not real
Check Question	**Check Answer**
• What do we mean by something being false?	• False or falsity means that what is thought or said contradicts reality

Fifth: Socratic Question	Typical Responses of Individuals
• Why is it important to objectively determine whether one's thinking/ ideas are true or false in reality?	• To communicate • To survive • To have a good life • To make sense of things

Check Question	Check Answer
• Why is it important to determine whether one's thinking/ideas are true or false in reality?	• Determining what is true or false leads to correctly identifying and understanding a reality, thinking and communicating clearly, and having a better life.

Step IV: Verification

Content Focus: Knowledge, Not Know, Not Sure	Understanding Goals
• A process of seeking verification or proving that what someone thinks, says, or experiences as being true or false in correspondence with, or in contradiction to reality, leads either to knowledge, not knowing, or not being sure • Knowledge, information, belief, or opinion are frequently used synonymously • Through verification, based upon proof, couples can understand the difference between knowledge, information, belief and opinion • Couples will learn how to determine the meaning of knowledge • Knowledge constitutes proof and leads to a correct identification of reality, where information, belief or opinion may or may not	• Thinking, interpreting, or saying something is true or false does not necessarily mean that it is; a rational and objective method of verification is required to determine whether our interpretation of reality leads either to knowledge, not knowing, or not being sure • They do not mean the same thing, however, people frequently do confuse the meaning of knowledge with that of information, belief, or opinion • Knowledge requires proof, and is obtained through a rational, objective methodology. • Information, belief and opinion only become knowledge when objectively proven to be true, or to correspond exactly to reality. Otherwise they are subject to doubt. Something thought to be knowledge (e.g. the earth is flat) and later proven false was never knowledge; rather it was a belief or opinion. • Knowledge is the result of consistently proving a correspondence between thought and reality • Our survival and quality of life are dependent upon distinguishing between what we know and do not know

First: Socratic Question	Typical Couple Response
• Given that an interpretation of a reality is either true or false, the problem is we do not _____ or have _____ as to whether it is correct or incorrect?	• Know, or knowledge

Check Question	Check Answer
• When we think, interpret, or say something is true or false, do we <u>know</u> whether it is what we think it <u>is</u>?	• Our thinking or interpretation may or may not tell us if something is true or false, therefore we need a rational and objective method of verifying whether what we think leads either to knowledge, not knowing, or not being sure

Second: Socratic Question	Typical Couple Responses
• Do knowledge, information, belief, or opinion mean the same thing?	• Yes • I don't know • I'm confused

Check Question	Check Answer
• Is knowledge the same as information, belief, or opinion?	• No, however, they are frequently used synonymously

Third: Socratic Question	Typical Couple Responses
• What is the one attribute or characteristic that differentiates knowledge from information, belief, or opinion?	• Evidence (practitioner: What is another word for evidence?) • Fact, factual (practitioner: How do you know it is factual?) • Proof (practitioner-probe for this answer)

Check Question	Check Answer
• How is knowledge different from information, belief, or opinion	• Knowledge requires proof, based upon evidence, whereas information, belief, and opinion do not. Knowledge is always true.

Fourth: Socratic Question	Typical Responses of Individual
• What is the meaning of the word knowledge?	• Something that is true • Something that can be proven • Something that is understood
Check Question	Check Answer
• How would you define knowledge?	• An interpretation that is proven to correspond to reality, and that is consistently true
Fifth: Socratic Question	Typical Responses of Individuals
• Why is it important to distinguish knowledge from information, belief, or opinion?	• To be objective in our thinking • To understand what we experience • To know what to do
Check Question	Check Answer
• Why distinguish knowledge from information, belief or opinion?	• In order to correctly identify reality, survive and to improve the quality of life

Practitioner's note:

- By seeking proof and verification for what we think, say, or experience that is not self-evident, we are pursuing a rational, non-contradictory methodology for determining what we know, don't know, or are not sure.
- The first four steps of the Conceptual Template have described a non-contradictory, rational, and objective approach to identifying a natural thinking process involved in the development and improvement of critical thinking skills.

The Universal Conceptual Template

Part Two: Application of a Rational Thinking Process (Steps V and VI)

Certain criteria and guidelines are essential for the effective application of Steps I–IV of the Conceptual Template in order to facilitate ethical development.

Determining what is important (values) to couples, both objectively and subjectively, provides them with a basis for their thinking regarding decisions, choices, and actions.

By learning how to evaluate objectively derived values and rights, couples can create a hierarchy upon which rational people could agree.

Evaluating criteria objectively will teach couples how to apply their critical thinking skills to making decisions, solving problems, or resolving conflict of either an ethical or non-ethical nature.

Step V: Criteria and Evaluation

Content Focus: Values and Rights	Understanding Goals

• The criteria we use in making one decision or choice over another is based upon what is important or of value to ourselves
 	
• The couples will learn how to determine the meaning of value or values
 	
• The couples will learn how to identify the purpose of values or the reason for values
 	
• It is necessary to have couples differentiate between objectively and subjectively derived values
 	
• It is because of life that values exist, therefore life is the highest value, and without life there would be no values
 	
• Survival and quality of life are greatly determined by the value people place on life
 	
• Freedom is the next highest value to life and health, and includes safety
 	
• Freedom requires that we recognize and respect everyone's values and rights
 	
• The couples will learn how to identify the meaning of rights
 	
• Rights have objective worth
 	
• Rights are the same as objectively derived values and also protect what people value subjectively
	• We have many different reasons why we make one decision or choice over another, however, it is what is important, or of <u>value</u> to us at a given time that determines what choice we make
	
	• A value is something that is important, that we want to attain, or keep
	
	• Values guide our thoughts and actions in both the moral and non-moral realm of experience
	
	• Objectively derived values are more important in reality because they are of value to all people for survival, improving or having a good life
	
	• Life is the highest value
	
	    • Without life values would not exist
	    • Life is the criterion by which values are judged
	    • Values are derived from and for human life
	
	• Valuing life is living life as you choose to, and/or in order to survive, have a good life, and to co-exist with others
	
	• Freedom is the next highest value for having a good life, because without freedom it would be difficult, if not impossible, to achieve other values
	
	• Freedom means that we can do whatever we choose as long as we do not infringe upon the higher, objectively derived values and rights of others
	
	• Rights are what people are entitled to, based upon objectively derived values
	
	• Rights are derived from what people objectively value in reality
	
	• Our objectively derived values are our rights; this also includes those things we value subjectively, as long as it does not infringe upon an objective, higher right of another/others

First: Socratic Question	Typical Responses of Individuals
• Why do we make one decision or choice over another?	• It's better • You like it • It's the right thing to do • It makes you feel good • To avoid trouble or conflict • To please others • You have to • You need to • You want to
Check Question	**Check Answer**
• How do people decide what choice or decision to make?	• What is important or of value to people determines what choice or decision they make

Practitioner's note:

• Once the couples respond as to why they make one choice over another, explain that all of their responses (better, need to, want to) are actually saying that they value one choice over another.

Second: Socratic Question	**Typical Responses of Individuals**
• How would you define "value"?	• Something that is important • Something that is moral • Something that is worthwhile • Something that is cherished
Check Question	**Check Answer**
• What do we mean by the word "value"?	• Something that is important, and worth attaining or keeping

Third: Socratic Question	**Typical Responses of Individuals**
• Why do we need values?	• To make choices • To make decisions • To determine right from wrong, or good from bad • To guide one's actions

Practitioner's note:

• If couples relate values to right or wrong, or good or bad, (morality, or ethics), then acknowledge that values can lead to a moral, or ethical base.

Check Question	Check Answer
• What is the purpose of values?	• Values give us direction in our thinking and guide us in our choices and actions

Practitioner's note:

- CT Values Identification Assignment (p.127)
- This assignment should be implemented before introducing the following FOURTH: Socratic Question.

Fourth: Socratic Question	Typical Responses of Individuals
• Which are more important: Objectively or subjectively derived values?	• Subjectively derived values • Objectively derived values

Check Question	Check Answer
• Are objectively or subjectively derived values more important?	• Objectively derived values are more important because they are essential to human life and well-being, while subjectively derived values are not

Practitioner's note:

- If there is confusion as to which is more important (objectively or subjectively derived values) go to Values Identification Assignment (p. 127) and implement number 5.

Fifth: Socratic Questions	Typical Responses of Individuals
• What is it that human beings value above all other values? • Why is life the highest value?	• Life • Without life there is nothing; without life there would be no other values

Practitioner's note:

- If couples respond with other than life, (e.g., freedom, air, water, etc.), determine if life is assumed

Check Question	Check Answer
• What is the highest value, and why?	• Life is the highest value, because without life there would not be any values

Sixth: Socratic Question	Typical Responses of Individuals
• What does it really mean to value life?	• Extremely varied

Practitioner's note:

- This is a good take home assignment.

Check Question	Check Answer
• What do you mean when you say you value life?	• Valuing life means living life as you would choose to while recognizing that life is the highest value

Check Question	Check Answer
• Other than valuing those things we need to survive, what is the next highest value?	• Freedom, because freedom allows us to make choices

Seventh: Socratic Question	Typical Couple Response
• Next to life and health, and those survival values such as air, water, shelter, etc., what is the most important value?	• Freedom • Safety • Security • Education of all types

Practitioner's note:

- If couples respond with safety or security, acknowledge that if those values are threatened they are not really free.
- It implies that safety and security are the result of being free.

Check Question	Check Answer
• Other than valuing those things we need to survive, what is the next highest value?	• Freedom, because freedom allows us to make choices

Practitioner's note:

- Based upon the Values Identification Assignment, have the couples create a hierarchy of their remaining objectively derived values.

Eighth: Socratic Question	Typical Responses of Individuals
• Does freedom mean that we can choose to do whatever we want?	• Yes; as long as no one is hurt • With reason (Clarify)

Practitioner's note:

- Distinguish between hurt, which may or may not affect a person's freedom, and harm, which always affects one's freedom.

Check Question	Check Answer
• If we are free, can we do whatever we choose?	• We can if we recognize and respect everyone's objectively derived higher values and rights

Ninth: Socratic Question	Typical Responses of Individuals
• Are rights derived from what we subjectively or objectively value in reality?	• Subjectively • Objectively

Check Question	Check Answer
• Are rights derived subjectively or objectively?	• Rights are derived objectively through a rational process of identifying reality

Tenth: Socratic Question	Typical Responses of Individuals
• What are "rights"?	• What we are entitled to • Freedom to have something • Privileges • They belong to everyone

Check Question	Check Answer
• What do we mean by "rights"?	• Something that we are entitled to, based upon an objectively derived hierarchy of values

Eleventh: Socratic Questions	Typical Responses of Individuals
• How do rights relate to values?	• Rights protect what people value • Rights and objectively derived values are the same • Everyone has a right to what is objectively of value

Check Question	Check Answer
• What is the relationship between rights and values?	• Objectively derived values and rights are the same, and subjectively derived values may or may not involve rights

Practitioner's note:

- Provide an example to determine if couples understand objectively derived values and rights; for example: is punctuality an objectively or subjectively derived value?

- Ask, "What does punctuality have to do with rights?"
- Answer

  - Punctuality is an agreement or contract.
  - By not being punctual, one is infringing upon a person's right to freedom, i.e., to make a different choice in terms of what one may have chosen to do if s/he would have known that the contract would be breached or broken.

Step VI: Judgment and Action

Content Focus: Morality and Justice	Understanding Goals
<ul><li>Moral conflicts involve a disagreement over rights, claims, or interests, what is right or wrong, or what is good or bad</li><li>The couples will learn how to determine the meaning of morality</li><li>In a conflict over rights, claims, or interests every rational person would want to be treated fairly, equitably, or in a just manner</li><li>The couples will learn how to determine the meaning of justice</li><li>Determining what is fair or just can both be achieved by applying an objective reasoning process (Steps 1–4) to what people can recognize and identify as their objectively derived values and rights</li></ul>	<ul><li>Disagreements involving people's rights, claims, or interests are moral conflicts</li><li>Morality is a code of values which guides our choices and actions in deciding what would benefit life and co-existence, while upholding our objectively derived values and inalienable rights</li><li>Even though not everyone may agree with the moral or ethical conclusion, each would agree that everyone has a right to be treated fairly and equitably; this leads to the idea of justice.</li><li>Justice is acknowledging everyone's human dignity and inalienable rights; justice is treating oneself and others in a way that rational human beings would agree is fair and equitable; justice is respecting and upholding truth and knowledge in relation to reality</li><li>By applying an objective reasoning process as described in the Conceptual Template (Steps 1–4) to what people can recognize and identify as their objectively derived values and rights (Step 5), people can achieve justice and fairness in thought, as well as in action (Step 6)</li></ul>

First: Socratic Question	Typical Responses of Individuals
• If people have a conflict involving rights, claims, or interest, what kind of conflict is it?	• Personal conflict • Values conflict • Conflict involving right and wrong • Moral conflict
Check Question	**Check Answer**
• What kind of conflicts involves peoples' rights, claims, interests, or what is right or wrong?	• Disagreements involving peoples' rights, claims, or interests are moral conflicts
Second: Socratic Question	**Typical Responses of Individuals**
• What do we mean by the word morality, or ethics?	• What people believe • What is right • A code for behavior, or code for living right
Check Question	**Check Answer**
• What do we mean by the word morality, or ethics?	• Morality is a code of values which guides our choices and actions in deciding what would benefit life and co-existence, while upholding our objectively derived values and inalienable rights
Third: Socratic Question	**Typical Responses of Individuals**
• Even though couples might disagree about what is moral or ethical everyone would want to be treated _____?	• Fairly • The same • As everyone else
Check Question	**Check Answer**
• Whether everyone agrees with the moral or ethical resolution to a conflict, how would everyone want to be treated?	• Everyone would agree that each person has a right to be treated fairly, or in a just manner

Fourth: Socratic Question	Typical Responses of Individuals
• What do we mean by the word justice?	• Treating everyone equally • Being fair • Respecting everyone's rights

Check Question	Check Answer
• What is justice?	• Justice is acknowledging everyone's human dignity and inalienable rights
	• Justice is treating oneself and others in a way that rational human beings would want to be treated
	• Justice is respecting and upholding truth, and knowledge of objectively derived values and rights, in relation to reality

Fifth: Socratic Question	Typical Responses of Individuals
• How do we determine and act upon what is fair or just?	• Apply the Golden Rule
	• Enact and enforce laws (religious and secular)
	• Establish rules

Check Question	Check Answer
• How can people achieve fairness and justice in their thinking, as well as in what they choose to do?	• People can learn to apply the objective reasoning process described in the Conceptual Template (Steps 1–4) to their objectively derived values and rights (Step 5), in order to better understand, resolve, and act upon, issues and conflict involving fairness and justice (Step 6)

Beyond the Six: Step Conceptual Template Principles and Justice

Practitioner's note:

• Once the Six-Step Conceptual Template has been understood, introduce the couples to a method of using a Principle to determine, that which is equitable or just when confronted with conflicting claims in a moral dilemma.

The Idea of Using a Principle for Solving Moral Dilemmas

A Principle does not mean, as in common usage, a strong moral conviction; nor is it a rule, which only works in specific situations.

A Principle is a standard, which provides a means for making an impartial or unbiased judgment. It equally preserves and protects the fundamental, natural, or universal rights of individuals. It also leaves open the possibility of coming to agreement through the guidance of rational standards, by which a judgment and its ensuing consequences can be deemed either beneficial or detrimental to human co-existence and happiness.

A Principle works across all situations, and must meet the criteria of reversibility and universalizability, which are explained as follows:

- Reversibility means that if, in a moral conflict, you do not know, in reality, which position you would be in, you would be willing to accept the (reverse) conditions or consequences of any of the possible positions.
- Universalizability is a check on reversibility. That is, any rational person would have to agree with the Principle being used, even if they personally or subjectively disagree, because, in reality, the Principle would be fair and equitable to everyone.

As moral conflict necessarily involves two or more people with two or more conflicting values, claims, or rights. If we were to put ourselves in the shoes of another, what would we think or value? (Use examples.) We would value that which the person in whose "shoes" we were standing valued. The conflict would not be resolved. Each time we take one position or another we are valuing, for that time, that position. The solution is to transcend all positions. That is, if we did not know which position we could be in, which position would we accept, or not accept as fair and equitable to everyone?

Reminder: This method of using reversibility and universalizability, and deriving a Principle on which to make judgments and take action, is based upon determining objectively derived values, as well as an objectively derived hierarchy of values (as in the Conceptual Template approach), and then applying them to the conflicting claims in the dilemma.

Applying the Idea of a Principle to a Moral Dilemma

Example

A person is rushing to someone who is choking to a hospital and s/he comes to a red traffic signal. *The driver stops, looks both ways, and sees that there is no traffic or pedestrians in any direction.* The driver must decide whether to run the red light, which is against the law, or wait for the light to change, which may endanger or end the life of the choking victim.

Dilemma Question

Should the driver break the law and run the red light in order to save the choking victim's life?

Method

(A)   Identify the parties involved in the dilemma:

1.   The choking victim
2.   The driver
3.   The Law (which represents individuals in society)

(B)   Questions:

1.   Would we want the driver to break the law and run the red light?

   i.   If we were the choking victim?
   ii. If we were the law (which represents individuals in society)?

2.   If we did not know which position we could be in, and we could be in any of the positions, what would we accept if we were being rational and objective about the circumstances or consequences?

(C)   Apply Reversibility and Universalizability

1.   Would the driver, or the law (which represents individuals in society) be willing to change places with the choking victim if the driver does not break the law and run the red light?

   i.   NO!
   ii. Because, neither the driver nor any other rational individual for whom the law exists would want the law to supersede the value of his/her life.

2.   Are all three positions Reversible and Universalizable?

   i.   NO!
   ii. Because, none of the three parties are willing to accept the conditions or consequences of the choking victim's position.

3.   Would the driver or the law (which represents individuals in society) change places with the choking victim if the driver does break the law and run the red light?

   i.   YES!
   ii. Because, the driver and the law (which represents individuals in society) would want to have their life valued above that of a law, which specifically prohibits going through a red light under any conditions, including the conditions stated in this example, in which a person is choking and the driver has taken all precautions regarding traffic and pedestrian safety.

4.   Are all three positions Reversible and Universalizable?

  i. YES!
  ii. Because, all three parties are willing to accept the conditions or consequences of the choking victim's position

(D) Deriving a Principle:

1. What Principle can be derived by applying Reversibility and Universalizability in this dilemma?
2. The Principle derived is that life has the highest value, and cannot be superseded by the law
3. As long as all precautions have been taken regarding the safety of other lives, all parties would

    i   Be willing to accept the conditions or consequences of any of the possible positions (Reversibility)
    ii   Agree with the Principle being used (Life has the highest value)
    iii Even if they subjectively disagree (Universalizability)

(E) Each Parties' objective responses to this dilemma:

1. Choking Victim – YES, the Driver should run the red light in order to save his/her life, which is of greater value than this particular law, under the stated conditions
2. Driver – YES, s/he should run the red light, because if s/he were in the position of the Choking Victim, s/he would want the value of his/her life to supersede this law, under the stated conditions
3. Law – YES, s/he should run the red light, because, even though the purpose of the law against running a red light is to protect life and maintain order, once that is done, as in the driver looking out for traffic and pedestrians.

    i. The law would recognize the Principle that life has a higher value than the specific law against running a red light
    ii. Also, individuals in society, for whom the law exists, would say YES, under the stated conditions, run the red light, because if they were in the position of the choking victim, they would objectively want the value of their life to supersede a specific law which prohibits running the red light, under any conditions

(F) Dilemma answers:

1. The driver should break the law and run the red light in order to save the choking victim's life, because rational and objective

people would agree that the value of one's life should supersede the letter of the law, namely, not running a red light under any conditions when the underlying Principle of the red light has been observed.

2. Based upon the principle that life has the highest value, the purpose of the law against running a red light is to protect human life, and is therefore derived from this principle.

Typical Exercise in Resolving a Moral Conflict

1. Present a moral/ethical problem and have the couple(s) discuss or write their solutions (do not emphasize Template)
2. Have the couple(s) review Template and concepts, then present the same moral dilemma or ethical problem again and have them apply the objective thinking process: The Conceptual Template

This exercise will result in one of the following possibilities:

1. Two objectively derived values or rights are involved and the couple (s) must determine which is the higher or more important value or right
2. An objectively derived value is opposed by a subjectively derived value and the couple(s) must determine that the objectively derived value supersedes the subjectively derived value
3. Two subjectively derived values are involved and couple(s) must determine that in reality, neither subjective value or claim supersedes the other; for example, one person wants to see movie A and the other wants to see movie B; both choices are subjective, therefore each has the right to make his/her own choice

---

Moral Conflict Diagram
Derived Values or Rights

1. **Objective/Objective = Moral/Ethical Dilemma**
2. **Objective/Subjective = Moral/Ethical Dilemma**
3. **Subjective/Subjective = No Moral/Ethical Dilemma**

Appendix

Objective Thinking Process Review

1. Review each step (I–VI) and all of the concepts.
2. Memorize the following:

   a   Steps I–VI
   b   The twelve concepts; and the order they appear in the conceptual framework
   c   The meaning and definition of each concept, and how they are connected.

A Daily Guide for Couples to Learning and Using the Six-Step Thinking Skills Program

1. Is what I am experiencing reality or my interpretation of reality?
2. Is what other(s) are experiencing reality or their interpretation?
3. Am I being objective or subjective in my thinking?
4. Are other(s) being objective or subjective in their thinking?
5. Is my interpretation correct (true) or incorrect (false)?
6. Are other(s) interpretation(s) correct (true) or incorrect (false)?
7. Do I know it, or is it a belief, opinion, or preference?
8. Does the other person(s) know it, or is it a belief, opinion, or preference?
9. Do I have evidence of proof or what I think?

   a   Have I tested the evidence?
   b   Does the other person(s) have evidence or proof?
   c   Have they tested it?

10. Do I know or not know, or am I not sure?
11. Does the other person(s) know or not know, or are they not sure?
12. What is important, or of value to me and the other person(s)?
13. Is what is being valued objective or subjective?
14. Is any one value of greater or lesser importance?
15. Is there a hierarchy of values?
16. Are my rights, and/or another's rights effected?
17. Can I determine which rights are of greater or lesser importance?
18. Is there a conflict of claims with another or others?
19. Can I determine what is fair and just for all parties involved?

20. What will be the consequences and/or results of my choices, decisions, and actions?

Part I: Learning and Understanding an Objective Thinking Process

EXERCISE #1 (Corresponds to Step 1 of the Six-Step Process)

Experiencing Reality (Corresponds to Step I).

(A) What is the reality that I am observing or experiencing?
(B) Describe your experience – do not interpret. Instruction: Observe what is being said by each person involved, in short, everything you notice. Descriptions only!

_____
_____
_____
_____
_____
_____

EXERCISE #2

Interpretation of Reality (Corresponds to Step II)

(A) What is your interpretation of what you have observed or experienced?
(B) Describe your initial thoughts, feelings and responses to what you have experienced.

_____
_____
_____
_____
_____
_____

EXERCISE #3 (Corresponds to Step III)

Question your interpretation:

(A) Is my interpretation of what I am observing and experiencing true (correct) or false (incorrect)?
(B) Am I being subjective, or am I being objective?
(C) Does my interpretation appear to correspond to reality? YES ———
     NO ———

_____
_____
_____
_____
_____
_____
_____

EXERCISE #4 (Corresponds to Step IV)

<u>Verifying</u> your interpretation of the reality perceived.

(A)   If your interpretation appears to correspond to reality, do you have evidence or proof?

    a   Describe the nature of your evidence and/or proof.
    b   Have you tested your evidence objectively?

(B)   If your interpretation does not appear to correspond to reality, which of the following should you do? (Choose those which best fit your situation).

    a   Seek more evidence/proof
    b   Draw conclusions
    c   Don't draw conclusions
    d   Ask for other's opinions
    e   Consider other possibilities
    f   Wait for change
    g   Test the evidence you have
    h   Other

(C)   Which of the following best describes your interpretation of the reality you have observed and experience (select one)?

    a   I know
    b   I don't know
    c   I'm not sure

_____
_____
_____
_____
_____
_____

Part II: Applying an Objective Thinking Skill Program to Issues, Decisions, Problems, and Choices

At this point some issues, conflicts, and/or problems can be resolved if you are able to objectively (evidence and testing) prove that you know or have knowledge of what you say or think. However, many situations will fall into the categories of not knowing, or not being sure, and you may be in a position where you will have to act, or make an important decision or choice. The following exercises are designed to provide you with guidelines for using the process learned in Steps I–IV, in order to have a reliable, objective basis for your actions, and/or decisions and choices.

EXERCISE # 5 (Corresponds to Step V)

Assessing criteria for evaluating what you think based upon Steps I–V.

Reminder: Values are guidelines for determining what is of greater or lesser importance, and for taking action.

(A)   What is being valued in the situation or problem? By you. By others.

(B)   Is what you or others are valuing objectively or subjectively derived?

(C)   If your answer is "objective," is there more than one value involved?

    a   NO

    b   If YES, how many? List below.

_____

_____

_____

_____

_____

_____

(D)   Create a hierarchy based upon what is objectively of greater or lesser importance.

_____

_____

_____

_____

_____

(E) Are there any rights involved? Yours and/or others? If so, list them below and form a hierarchy as in D above.

_____

_____

_____

_____

_____

_____

Comment: At this point, if you are continuing to be objective in your thinking, you will have a rational-moral basis for making a choice, or decision, or taking an action.

Question: Does your issue, problem, and/or decision involve a question of what is moral (right or wrong, good or bad)?

1. NO
2. NOT SURE
3. YES

If you answered YES, go on to Step VI. If you answered NO, stop here; you should be able to identify and objectively understand and/or resolve what you are questioning and/or experiencing. If you're NOT SURE, go back and review Steps I–V, and work through exercises 1–5.

Values Identification Assignment

Step V Criteria and Evaluation (See page 115 in this manual for reference)

1. Have the couple as a pair (or as individuals depending on the practitioner's approach) make a list of those things that they value.
2. Then have the couple as a pair (or as individuals depending on the practitioner's approach) separate both of their lists of values into the two following categories:

    a Those values that all rational people would consider necessary to one's existence, well-being, or happiness, whether they are aware of it or not.
    b Those values that would be important to some individuals, but would not be important to all rational people.

3. Have the couple as a pair (or as individuals depending on the practitioner's approach) suggest three–four values from both categories and write them on a separate list.

Note: Review at this time the meaning and differences between subjectivity and objectivity.

4. Then have the couple as a pair (or as individuals depending on the practitioner's approach) separate the suggested values into categories A or B. (This can be achieved by having the couples apply Steps I–IV of the Conceptual Template in order to determine whether a given value is important to some people (subjectively derived), or needed by all people (objectively derived), based upon reality.*)

QUESTION IN STEP V

5. Have couple select one value from each category (A and B) and ask them to determine which value is more important. (Repeat this exercise until they understand clearly that objectively derived values are more important than subjectively derived values because they are based upon reality.)

GENERAL QUESTIONS

1. Describe what you think it means to value "life."
2. Define what freedom means to you.
3. List some rights you feel you have.

    a   Why do you have these?
    b   Can they be "taken away"?

4. Have the couple discuss whether they feel rights are cultural, or bound to a historical time period.
5. Do rights change?

SPECIFIC DISCIPLINE QUESTIONS

Each discipline treats how they view people differently, and you can relate the question of values and rights to this. For example, in science if testing a new drug on a human is more effective than testing on mice, can a scientist select humans and experiment? Why or why not?

There are many obvious examples involving human rights in all disciplines throughout history. The practitioner can select whatever s/he chooses and present the situation as rights in conflict to turn the discussion to this step of the template.

Needs are used here in their metaphysical sense; i.e., that which is objectively important, natural or innate, or universal to human beings; not that which is particular or subjective to the individuals' well-being.

EXERCISE #6 (Corresponds to Step VI)

Judgment and Action: Determining what is fair and choosing to act upon it.

(A) Is there a conflict of claims and/or interests with another or others? Explain and/or describe below.
(B) Have all parties' values and rights been considered objectively in Steps (exercises) I–V? Have they been put in order of objective importance?
(C) Using the objective thinking process in Steps I–IV, and taking into account what is being valued by all parties (Step V), including the organization of a hierarchy of values and rights, determine a fair and equitable solution for resolving the issues and/or conflicts you are experiencing.
(D) Given that reasonable people can disagree, what you want to determine in this exercise is that which everyone can rationally agree to as being objectively fair and just, even though they may personally (subjectively) disagree.

_____
_____
_____
_____
_____
_____

Step VI: Judgment and Action or Ethics and Justice: General Questions

1. Have the couple as a pair (or as individuals per practitioner's process) describe what they believe it means to be "treated fairly."

    a Have the couple as a pair (or as individuals per practitioner's process) discuss the question, "How does the concept of fairness affect our rights?"

b   Have the couple as a pair (or as individuals per practitioner's process) list their code of values in regards to being treated fairly as well as treating others fairly.

c   Have the couple as a pair (or as individuals per practitioner's process) indicate which beliefs are unique to them personally, or are held by a society or culture, and again indicate if that society or culture may be unique to an individual.

2.   Have the couple as a pair (or as individuals per practitioner's process) make a list of five topics or situations which they believe would constitute an ethical dilemma.

a   Write each topic on an individual sheet of paper for the couple.

b   (Applies only to group therapy.) The practitioner can collect these the next day, select some and give to another couple to adjudicate, using the steps of the template.

c   Have the couple as a pair (or as individuals per practitioner's process) indicate what they would have to learn to resolve the problem, since some topics might require information one or both individuals of the couple wouldn't possess.

d   Have the couple as a pair (or as individuals per practitioner's process) provide their opinions on what is the role of power or authority in enforcing ethics?

*Practitioner's note: This is an opportunity to review the thinking/reasoning process per individual and the corresponding moral cognitive stage.

Six Stages of Moral Reasoning

In the late 1950s, Lawrence Kohlberg began to collect data related to moral questions. Kohlberg had studied Jean Piaget's earlier work in cognitive and moral development and used this as a foundation for a longitudinal study of moral reasoning. Piaget's work focused primarily on uncovering cognitive[1] stages.[2] Kohlberg's study also focused on a developmental sequence of stages and revealed that individuals restructure their thinking about social and moral questions just as they develop their cognitive structure from the very concrete toward the more abstract.

Specifically, Kohlberg introduced a developmental theory for moral reasoning. The theory describes six stages of moral reasoning.[3]

Table 11.1 Sequence and Explanation of Kohlberg's Six Stages of Moral Judgment/Reasoning

LEVEL I   Pre-Conventional

At this level the child is responsive to cultural rules and labels of good and bad, right and wrong, but interprets these labels in terms of either the physical or the hedonistic consequences of action (punishment, reward, exchange of favors) or in terms of the physical power of those who enunciate the rules and labels. The level is divided into two stages.

- Stage 1: Punishment and obedience orientation.

  - The physical consequences of action determine its goodness or badness regardless of the human meaning or value of these consequences.
  - Avoidance of punishment and unquestioning deference to power are valued in their own right, not in terms of respect for an underlying moral order supported by punishment and authority (the latter being Stage 4).

- Stage 2: Naively egoistic orientation.

  - Right action consists of that which instrumentally satisfies one's own needs/desires and occasionally those of others.
  - Human relations are viewed in terms of the marketplace.
  - Thus, while elements of fairness, reciprocity, and equal sharing are present, they are always interpreted in a physical or pragmatic way, that is, reciprocity is a matter of "you do something for me and I'll do something for you."

Note: Pre-conventional Stages 1 and 2 are the early stages of cognitive-moral development in children. These stages when occurring in adulthood are indicative of inadequate development.

LEVEL II   Conventional

At this level, maintaining the expectations of the individual's family, group, or nation is perceived as valuable in its own right, regardless of immediate and obvious consequences. The attitude is not only one of conformity to personal expectations and social order, but of loyalty to it, of actively maintaining, supporting, and justifying the order and of identifying with the persons or group involved in it. At this level there are two stages:

- Stage 3: Good-boy or nice-girl orientation

  - Ethical decisions are based on what pleases, helps, or is approved of by others

- Stage 4: Law and order orientation

  - This stage is oriented toward authority, fixed rules, and the maintenance of the social order
  - Right behavior consists of doing one's duty, showing respect for authority and maintaining the given social order for its own sake

Table 11.1 (Cont.)

LEVEL III   Post-Conventional

At this level moral/ethical value resides in conformity by the self to shareable standards, rights, or duties.

- Stage 5: Social-contract legalistic orientation

    - Recognition of an arbitrary element or starting point in rules or expectation for the sake of agreement
    - Duty is defined in terms of contract, general will, or rights of others, and majority will and welfare

- Stage 6: Conscience or principle orientation

    - Orientation not only to actually ordained social rules, but to principles of choice involving logical universality and consistency
    - These are universal principles of justice, of the reciprocity and equality of human rights, and of respect for the dignity of human beings as individual persons

These six stages represent patterns of thinking/reasoning which integrates each person's experience and perspective on specific moral issues. Although everyone may be able to memorize certain civic virtues/values, not everyone will think about important issues in the same way or act according to the same "learned" virtues/values. Therefore, rather than to teach the moral rule related to a specific situation, practitioners can help couples examine the reasoning used to solve moral problems. Practitioners can help couples examine their own moral reasoning and the reasoning of others through the understanding and application of specific and essential philosophical concepts of human thought described in the Conceptual Template Program (CT).

Glossary

The meaning of each of the following terms is based upon an operational definition; that is, an agreed upon or common understanding of the meaning of a term or concept (idea) used by people to communicate or understand what is experienced.

The definitions are presented in the order in which they appear in the Practitioners Instructional Manual.

Reality: That which exists, or the nature of things.
Nihilism: A form of skepticism, which denies that reality exists.
Illusion: A misperception of reality based upon a desire or wish for something to be that is not.
Life (Human): The condition of existing, as a self-generated, self-sustaining organism with the rational capability to govern one's own will or consciousness.
Nature of Things: The process by which things function and exist.

Actuality: An individual or group's interpretation of a specific reality.

Subjectivity: Basing what one holds to be true or false on one's feelings or interpretations alone, rather than upon the attributes of the object itself or of the reality being considered.

Objectivity: Focusing upon the attributes or characteristics of the object itself or the reality being considered; it excludes desires in considering the truth.

True or Truth: A thought or statement that corresponds to reality.

False: A thought or statement that contradicts reality.

Proof: Objective evidence of the validity or truth establishing actual correspondence of the reality being considered.

Verification: The rational process to establish/validate the truth, accuracy, or reality of a thought, statement, or condition.

Methodology: The study of the principles or procedures of inquiry in a particular field.

Knowledge: Proven correspondence between thought and reality.

Opinion/Belief: Holding or thinking something to be either true or false, qualified by uncertainty or doubt, because the truth or falsity, with regard to the actual or real, is either not proven or not provable.

Non-Contradictory: A thought, statement, or action that consistently corresponds to the truth or a particular reality.

Critical Thinking Skills: The ability to develop and apply a logical, rational process of thought which allows one to look at ideas and issues objectively.

Hierarchy: Placing things in order of importance.

Value(s): Something that is important or have worth. Guidelines for one's choices or actions.

Rights: A just or lawful claim, based upon objectively derived values and objective hierarchy of values; i.e., life (and its sustaining physical and metaphysical needs), freedom, health, and education, which cannot rationally be infringed upon or denied.

Metaphysical: Pertaining to reality, existence, or the nature of things.

Conflict: A disagreement between two or more people involving a difference of beliefs, opinions, ideas, or interests.

Morality: A code of values which guides one's choices and actions in deciding that which benefits life and co-existence.

Moral Conflict: A disagreement over conflicting rights, justice concerns, or what is right or wrong, good or bad pertaining to life or co-existence.

Inalienable Rights: A just or lawful claim, which is derived from one's existence; a metaphysical fact of reality, which rationally cannot be infringed upon or denied.

Ethics: The science or study of morality that deals with discovering and defining a rational and objective means of determining that which benefits life and co-existence, and is fair, equitable, or just.

Fairly: Treating everyone in an equitable and just manner.

Justice: Respecting and upholding truth, and knowledge of objectively derived values and rights in relation to reality.

Fundamental: Pertains to a person's right to his/her own life, from which all other rights are derived.

Rules: Guidelines for governing individual and/or societal action and behavior in specific situations.

Principle: A standard, which provides a means for making an impartial or unbiased judgment. It equally preserves and protects the fundamental, natural, or universal rights of individuals. It also leaves open the possibility of coming to agreement through the guidance of rational standards, by which a judgment and its ensuing consequences can be deemed either beneficial or detrimental to human co-existence and happiness. As used herein, a principle does not mean, as in common usage, a strong conviction with regard to a particular moral issue, but rather a "rule" which meets the criteria of reversibility and universalizability.

Conviction: A firm or strongly held belief or opinion.

Reversibility: In a moral conflict all parties would be willing to agree upon a judgment or decision when they trade places with others in the situation being judged.

Universalizability: A check on reversibility. Even though they might subjectively disagree, objectively all parties would agree to be bound by the condition that all judgments are to apply consistently to everyone in a similar situation(s).

Moral Dilemma: A conflict between two or more individuals over rights, interests, or claims.

Chapter 12

Transcript of Author Teaching the Conceptual Template

The following is a transcription of the author teaching the Conceptual Template process (CT) to a licensed professional practitioner. It is intended to be a complimentary companion to this book's Instructional Manual, demonstrating what this approach can "look like" in a real-world, clinical setting. Because the nature of these essential concepts and their interrelationships can be complex, particularly with regards to morality and fairness or justice concerns, it is suggested that this method of counseling is most helpful to couples when it is used in a more informal and down to earth manner. As the philosopher Trungpa (1973) suggested, in more words or less, "You can go to the top of the mountain but you must put your feet on the ground."

Each session herein is longer in length than a typical session in a clinical setting. Five to ten psychotherapy sessions would correspond to one session as described herein, which last for several hours each, and in this example involves an individual familiar with much of the content.

The transcript covers multiple sessions where the teacher illuminates why the CT can be a beneficial tool for the couple therapist, by either implicitly or explicitly relating how the practitioner could adopt and integrate specific CT constructs into their practice. Session 1 is an introduction and orientation for the couple when first meeting with the therapist. This orientation is not transcribed but is discussed and outlined in **Session 1** below (pp. 141–142). The introduction to this approach should be flexible as to the clinician's background, knowledge of Kohlberg's theory of moral development, cognitive and cognitive-moral stage development, as well as clinical experience. As such the author is suggesting that the content of the first session be left to the provider's discretion based upon their professional experience. Nevertheless, that which the author considers to be important issues for the first session is outlined in the orientation.

At the beginning of Session 2, Part 1 (pp. 142–158), the author asks the couple what they understood from the first session's orientation. In the transcript this question is asked as follows: *"How do you understand what we were talking about at our first meeting?"* This affords both the therapist and the couple opportunity to clarify any questions or possible misunderstanding. Once these concerns have been discussed and the couple understands more fully this approach, then the assignment given to the couple at the close of the first session is addressed, namely, "What is meant by the term reality and why is it important to understand reality?" This is a critical juncture; it is important for the therapist as well as the couple to understand that the CT approach is not in any manner or form saying, suggesting or implying what reality is per se. The CT 's sole purpose is to encourage autonomy in one's use of their own faculty of reason, mindfully using the naturally occurring and essential concepts our mind innately has at its disposal to determine, check and countercheck, both our capability to understand reality and also to then respond in a non-contradictory and objective manner, both in the non-moral and moral domain of human experience.

Consistent with this aim, the term reality is defined by the couple through "Socratic" questioning and dialogue and if necessary didactically refined by the practitioner. The term "reality" can be defined in a way that would be difficult if not impossible from a rational objective perspective to find disagreement, because of its neutrality, it cannot be reduced further, or because it is axiomatic; reality is operationally defined then as, "It is what it is" or "It is whatever it is," "Reality is what is" (Aristotle, 1952). This definition can be extrapolated to that which exists or the nature of things (Aristotle, Plato). There is not a rational argument in this definition because no one is saying what any particular reality is; it is merely being asked, "What does the *term* reality mean?" that is, when we use this word what are we meaning by the term itself. As earlier paraphrased, "If words do not have a particular meaning, then there is no conscious conceptual meaning which humans could use in order to communicate and construct meaning (Aristotle, 1952, p. 525). This modus operandi appears unique to humans, by means of our faculty of reason, in both determining and responding to reality. Other than our autonomic nervous system (that which happens automatically, like our cardiovascular or endocrine system) or our will to survive, and to improve, or to have a better or good life, the CT is purely a method representative of the means by which our ability to comprehend realities is determined by reason, forming mental connection between innate and universal essential concepts humans have for the purpose of understanding and constructing meaning of experience.

Therefore, during Session 2 the couple through Socratic questioning and didactic refinement defines the meaning of the term reality as "What is." The couple then begins to identify, define and interrelate several essential concepts naturally used in comprehending their experience of reality. The essential concepts/ideas discovered or brought to the foreground of conscious-awareness by the couple through collaborative effort with the guidance of the therapist during Session 2, Part 1, include: perception/interpretation, true, false, objectivity, subjectivity. These concepts along with those that follow in Session 2, Part 2, Session 3 and 4, all can help the couple to better understand reality and the potential to improve their interaction and mindful communication, particularly in regard to resolving conflict in a just manner.

At the beginning of Session 2, Part 2 (pp. 158–172) there is a teacher's review. Then the foundation that has been being built by the earlier defined and interrelated essential concepts are connected through understanding their interrelationships to the essential concept of *knowledge*. Knowledge is differentiated from perception or an interpretation of a reality as well as in contradistinction to an opinion or belief. Proof or objective proof is discussed as the criterion of knowledge. Distinguishing knowledge from interpretation, belief, and opinion is critically important in that perception, as understood and stated in the marketing world, "Perception is reality" to the consumer (people). This confusion of perception, opinion, or belief as being knowledge or understanding a reality creates unnecessary conflict in couples' relationships or interactions in general. Lastly, the importance of the concept of value in guiding one's action is discussed within the context of objectively derived values (based upon needs, both physical and metaphysical) being distinguished from subjectively based values (personal wants/desires).

In Session 3 (pp. 173–184) Stages of moral development are clinically explored. A specific moral dilemma is presented and suggested as a means to clinically evaluate couples with regard to their being Conventional (Stages 3 and 4), relativistic, or Post-conventional (Stage 5 or 6) in their stage of moral judgment/reasoning. Clinically explaining stages of moral development can provide the practitioner who may not be familiar with Kohlberg's stages a sense of their development that is easily understood relative to those described from empirical research. The clinical explanation in a simplified form also can give the practitioner a gestalt of moral development. The value of a clinical measurement gives the practitioner a clearer sense of whether or not the goal of moral development is being achieved during couple counseling.

The Session 4 (pp. 184–197) introduces the essential concept of rights as related to values and morality. Again this is creating a connection or interrelatedness to previous concepts such as values or in particular objectively derived values to rights and rights to values or in terms of moral reasoning/judgment, conflicting interests or rights. As in each session, when interconnecting each concepts it is constructing, somewhat visually, the ultimate goal, which is being consciously aware of the CT. The fifth and final session relates to the earlier concepts to how to determine what is fair or just. Role taking (Selman) is indicated as part of this process as is empathy. The veil of ignorance (Rawls, 1971, pp. 136–142) and "moral musical chairs" (personal communication, Kohlberg) are explained such that it can serve as a guide to couples in determining that which is just in couples having a conflict of interests or rights.

This transcript's intent is to show that a CT approach to couple counseling is of value. It encourages a more general, although clear understanding of the essential philosophical concepts and their interrelationships such that the therapeutic relationship is to some degree a dialogue. Even if presented in a somewhat dialectical manner, it is of lesser importance to be overly linear or didactic.

These essential ideas/concepts are used by us all, even if we are not consciously aware or mindful of them in our everyday experiences, communication, or, in general, our lives. The concepts are universal and, in some ways, familiar, perhaps so common, that we can lose sight of their essential meaning and significance. Therefore, the practitioner should allow for a breadth of latitude or openness in how each of us individually, or as a couple in a relationship, brings this conceptual awareness to conscious awareness.

Session 1: Orientation and Introduction

Defining the Concepts of True and False. Objectivity and Subjectivity

SESSION 1: ORIENTATION

The first session is somewhat of an informal discussion with regard to the orientation that will be used in couple counseling. There is a general overview of the Conceptual Template. The overview does not and should not use any of the essential concepts in its explanation. It is explained, however, that there are essential concepts that our mind naturally uses to understand our experiences (of reality). The couple is told that this approach will assist them to identify, define, and to interrelate these ideas for themselves. In this way they are not being told what to think, how to think, or what they should think. Discovering this for themselves, through their own naturally occurring reasoning/cognitive process and ability, they can then determine for themselves the value of what they have learned using the Conceptual Template itself. There is additionally a very brief overview of cognitive and cognitive-moral development. This includes two cognitive stages (Piaget, 1932) such as concrete and formal operational reasoning; these cognitive stages are suggested, as they are the most readily relatable to adults, particularly when given a simple example of the difference(s). It is explained, in a simplified manner, that concrete reasoning is thinking in black or white terms and formal operational reasoning is thinking in terms of possibilities. An example can be given, such as comparing a mechanic who is concrete operational having difficulty with solving a mechanical problem because s/he can only approach the concern in one way, with a formal operational mechanic that can think of other possibilities to solve the problem. It is also indicated that people can be concrete in one area of their life and formally in another domain. For example a neurosurgeon, when doing brain surgery thinks in possibilities, but how s/

he relates to their partner can be in black or white terms. Lastly, Kohlberg's empirical stages of moral development are outlined or described so the couple can understand to some degree how structural development occurs, and can also relate to these stage orientations. They are then given an assignment for session 2 to define the term reality. It is emphasized that it is not being asked either how they understand, nor for any form of explanation of reality, namely, their metaphysical perspective, but rather, it is being asked for a definition of the meaning of the term reality, so that we are all on the same page so to speak; they can use any resource. As part of this assignment they are also asked: "Why is it important to understand reality?" The first session closes with questions or concerns, which, the couple may want to have addressed.

SESSION 2, PART 1: DEFINING THE MEANING OF THE TERM REALITY AND THE INITIAL ESSENTIAL CONCEPTS AND ISSUES USED FOR UNDERSTANDING REALITY: ACTUALITY (PERCEPTION/INTERPRETATION), TRUE AND FALSE, OBJECTIVITY AND SUBJECTIVITY

(T) = Teacher
(P) = Practitioner

(T): Can you state your name and what you do?
(P): I am a Behavioral Health Specialist at a High School, working mainly with teenagers for the past eighteen years. My degree is in social work; I have a Masters in Social Work. I also started my private practice just a few years ago and have a license in clinical social work.
(T): Ok. The way I would normally begin is how I began with you last week *or how you might begin with a client or couple. We* discussed in general and informally, *what we would be doing in this process and* the purpose of the CT. The second time I see a couple, I would begin as we are doing today, by asking them: *"How do you understand what we were talking about at our first meeting?"* Since you learned this eighteen years ago, how do you sort of remember what this is all about?
(P): I remember this was about learning how to think; how do we think clearly about what we see and what reality is, versus what our interpretations are of reality.
(T): Good, so then we are going to be talking about reality. I then ask, in one form or another, whether teaching a practitioner, counseling couples, or a client the following: *"Why do you think it is important that we might talk about reality?"*
(P): I may use different words for it. But, it is important because a lot of the time the clients feel or think that what they are thinking or feeling is real, but it could be a misinterpretation of experiences. So they could see things and then think that something is happening but it really isn't what is going on because it is based on what they are experiencing.

(T): Could you give me an example of something like that in your experiences in couple counseling, where that was the case?

(P): Yeah! A lot of times, if the male feels like they, that the wife does not give them enough sex, then they feel like the wife doesn't love them anymore. And then, it starts to go on this tangent, where I guess they start thinking or feeling like they are not valued or their wife doesn't care about them, just because the physical part is not there.

(T): Is that a common issue?

(P): Yeah.

(T): And, that could be a misinterpretation?

(P): Yeah. And it might be important for them to identify that that is not the correct interpretation.

(T): Can you explain why that might be important or of value for them to become aware that it may be a misinterpretation?

(P): Yeah. Because a lot of times they feel unloved if that happens, and they get resentful. Instead of trying to communicate their resentment, which they might not even know that their feeling that way, they are just upset and the problems continue. And it gets worse between the two of them because they are not communicating what they're feeling, what they are thinking. So, instead of asking the wife, "Do we not have sex anymore? Do you not love me or do you not care about me?" or whatever it is, he makes up stories in his head about what the wife is thinking or feeling and then that causes him to feel, you know, resentful, and then maybe to do things that are unhealthy within the marriage.

(T): So then it is important to understand reality in this kind of circumstance so there can be a clear kind of communication about what he is feeling and what she is thinking or feeling so that they can better understand one another.

(P): Yeah, right.

(T): Rather than going down some track that might be harmful, that is, a misinterpretation. Yes. Am I right?

(P): Yes.

(T): Ok. So, the first concern is *REALITY*.

(P): Ah hum.

(T): We are trying to identify reality, and that is a good example, of, that is the reality. The second thing is we need to look at or be aware of is, *we experience reality* whatever that may be. For example, this man is experiencing something with his wife, and *that is reality that he is experiencing it.*

(P): Right.

(T): But that is not the issue right? Because in reality we can only experience what, when we are experiencing?

(P): What do you mean?

(T): It wasn't an easy question! The only thing we can experience, is what, at any time?

(P): That we are experiencing through the senses?

(T): Right. The only thing we experience is what? What comes through the senses, has to be what, unless there is something wrong with the senses? What comes in through the senses? What are we are always experiencing? Like what are you experiencing right now?

(P): That I know that are coming through my brain, the signals that are coming through my brain? (Laughter) I don't know. That is coming from what?

(T): Through your senses, which is what?

(P): Reality?

(T): Yeah, so the only thing we experience is reality.

(P): Yeah.

(T): Now as we experience reality the only thing the senses absorb is what is, which is what exists, in whatever form that may be. It could be then misinterpreted. The brain is interpreting all those things coming through the senses. So, reality is what we are experience. *It is important for an individual or couple to understand that, that what we are trying to understand is, reality.* And, therefore), w*e need to understand what we mean by the term reality.*

  So if you had to define the term reality, which is also what you would then ask the client(s) at this juncture, is: How would you define the meaning of the word reality?

(P): Reality is what is.

(T): (Then it would be asked) *"Why do you think it is important that we talk about reality?"* They may respond in a little different way than you did. They might say, well it is important for us to understand reality because ... what might an individual or couple say? Why is it important to understand reality?

(P): In order that we know what is going on. So you know, something that we can agree on in that, because, it is what it is, right?

(T): So that is basic. And that makes sense. It is pretty hard to disagree, if a person even said what you said, "reality is what it is." It is very hard to disagree and this is very important for a practitioner to know that (or a couple to understand). *By saying reality is whatever it is, or reality is what it is, is not saying what it is; that is where the conflict can arise. But we cannot disagree that whatever it is, it is what it is.* And in fact, *it is sometimes important to explain that how we might perceive a reality or how another animal or insect or what have you perceives realities, they also have to perceive reality, because if they didn't perceive reality correctly, just like us, if we don't perceive or interpret a reality correctly, what can happen to us, in reality?*

(P): We could die.

(T): Yeah, we could die. Sometimes that is hard to get people to say. People don't like to think about death. At least that is what I *believe* is the reason. People sometimes just do not want to say that. So you want them to realize that; it is that important. *If we don't understand the reality, we could die.*

(P): Right.

(T): So, to go back again to what we were talking about ... is that if we don't understand reality like you said, we could die and so it somehow makes me wonder personally why we aren't more conscious of those kinds of things. We also don't think a lot about, "What is the reality?" We just think because we think something that is the way it is. As Sigmund Freud said "The greatest cathexis is to one's self." We get away with a lot of it, but sometimes we don't. Sometimes people die because of not correctly identifying it. But, it is that significant, and in a relationship it is no different. If there is not an understanding of the reality the main problem as you said is, they can't communicate. Or if they do communicate, it is not going to be about reality; it is about something, that is, as you put it, that they are interpreting to be reality. Also as you said, if they are having an issue where the husband feels that his wife doesn't love him because she is not having enough sex with him or what have you, then that is a miscommunication and he can think all kinds of things and that can snow ball into something a lot more difficult. *So, the bottom line is, the first thing we need to do in any kind of communication is to understand the reality.*

(P): Right.

(T): Now we are not always going to understand reality. Sometimes we are going to misunderstand the reality, just like the example.

(P): Right. Even in counseling if the husband says we're not having enough sex, the counselor can interpret that as they're not having sex at all, but in reality they could be having it maybe twice a week which is normal, maybe it's not, I don't know, you know, so...

(T): Right.

(P): We're not specific about it. What the reality is, is their situation, and as a practitioner you can also misinterpret the situation.

(T): Correct, very good. You make a very good point. And, a part of this, that when you're doing this, as a therapist, is your interpretation, of what somebody is saying, (facial expressions, etc.) So, let's say they said, he said, well, we have sex twice a week; I don't feel like she really loves me. And she says, well I didn't know that you felt that way. And let say they already have a couple of children, and she says, you know when I come home from work I am very tired, and you want to have sex right away, and I am just tired. It has nothing to do ... right ... so now he is hearing that, that doesn't end the issue necessarily.

(P): Right.

(T): So now that dialogue has to go on between them. What do they mean? For one person, that interpretation is, that is a lot of sex, like to her, because she is saying I am tired.

(P): Right.

(T): Ok. Good. So, if they do not communicate about that in a way, they both understand, what they mean, they still...

(P): I mean their feelings are still there. I mean they're both resentful because life is hard because she comes home, she takes care of the kids, and her priorities are probably the kids. She has to cook, clean and all that stuff. You know, her priority is not to have sex during the week or whatever.

(T): That may be true. I mean you said that is true. My experience as a therapist is the case that women often feel, particularly today, it is different than the 1950s when women's social role identity was one of being the housewife or the caregiver, nurturer. They felt that was their obligation. I'll give you an example of that. I was once going to (was at a wedding). There was a woman I was talking to at the home where I was staying, who I didn't know. She had 10 children.

(P): My gosh!

(T): I wasn't yet a psychologist and was a little more naive than I am today. But I said to her, I don't know why anybody would say this, but I did, I said "You must have a pretty good marriage, having had ten children." She then got really upset, not at me, and said, what are you talking about. My husband came home drunk every night, had sex with me, and I had ten children one year after the next after the next; I can't stand him. So even the therapist can misperceive, misinterpret, or misunderstand what another person is experiencing. So we always want to be aware as a therapist as practitioners of any kind, that everybody is in their own mind, and if we do not understand what that is, we are not going to be able to communicate as well.

(P): Right.

(T): Some things are self-evident other things are not. So that is why you want to begin with the concept, not the concept, excuse me, with the *term reality*. Do you think reality is a concept, just out of curiosity?

(P): Well what do you mean by concept?

(T): A concept is a construct about something. Like if I say this is a clock, the construct is clock.

(P): Yeah.

(T): You do? Ok, it might be important to understand that reality just is. A construct about reality is something else. So, we'll get to that. We *are interpreting* and we understand why that is so important. And, we understand that is important to each individual you are working with. The other thing that you always want to be conscious of is, whatever we're thinking, the other person may understand or not. Or whatever we're thinking about whatever the other person is thinking we don't have a clue, necessarily. And so it is an important concept. And so now we're *interpreting as the next step.* We are experiencing reality and you said that then we interpret it (reality) and that is the next step. Right? We had a term for that when first learned, 18 years ago and the reason we used that term we gave a name to that. Do you remember what that was?

(P): Yeah, *Actuality.*

(T): Yeah, actuality, and the reason we used that term is that it came out of something historical and that is why I used it (Krishnamurti). But we could also say we form a *construct.* That would be another way to put it. Whatever it is, (the term used) it is *our interpretation* of that *reality.* So that actuality, whatever we are interpreting, has to be, and again, like when you are working with a person, you would do the same thing. You are sort of guiding them in a way. You are really trying to be Socratic and ask them questions, but sometimes you have to do it in a way that the concept(s) seem self-evident. For example, if I were to say to you, you are interpreting something, so your interpretation of whatever it is, has to be either ___blank___ or ___blank___? And people might have trouble with that (difficulty with the framing of the question in this manner). But when you are saying that "It is either blank or blank, it has to be either what or what?"

(P): You are asking me?

(T): Yes.

(P): True or False.

(T): Yeah. Some people might say correct or incorrect. But we will use the concepts true or false ... I usually just draw this nut shaped thing (line) around *Actuality* (our interpretation*) and True.* And if you ask me, it is a pretty interesting metaphor. That is what people usually do. Why might I have done that?

(P): Because, if our actuality is true then it correlates to reality.

(T): Well that may be one reason. That is not the reason though. Why might I do that? That is not something you should particularly know. I just do it so that people do realize it.

(P): Realize what?

(T): Something about, why would I maybe do that, draw (a line) around true and actuality? What you said was really pretty good. I could use that. But, there is another reason I might do that.

(P): I don't know.

(T): Could you guess?

(P): Why would you draw a circle (somewhat shaped like a cashew nut) around actuality and true?

(T): Yes.

(P): Just to make us think a little bit harder (Laughter) about it?

(T): Maybe.

(P): Yeah, anything. And figure it out, how do we know that it is true?

(T): That might be a pretty good idea. Right?

(P): Right.

(T): That might be a reason, any other possible reason? That was a good one. I never had anybody say that!

(P): I don't know.

(T): Well, the reason is, and the reason somebody pointed out that it is nut shaped, is it looks like a nut. It looks a little bit like a cashew (Laughter). Yeah, does it or not?

(P): (Laughter) *Not really!*

(T): *So, our Actuality or interpretations, constructs) are different* (More laughter). What do you think it looks like?

(P): It looks like a brain. (Laughter)

(T): Oh, it looks like a brain. Yeah, that's right, right? So here again we can see that what I say and what you perceive or hear or see is different than what I am. Even the brain is a good idea. So, we say that is the brain. So, then you want to bounce off what that person is saying to you, hearing them, acknowledging, and communicating. And I would take (use) that if they said that. I have never had anybody say that. So, I would just say, if teaching you as a couple, I would say, "Oh you think it looks like a brain?" So, brain and true, and I am perceiving reality and my brain says true. What might you think the reason that I might do that? Because?

(P): It is true.

(T): Because it is true?

(P): Yeah, I already said that.

(T): The brain is perceiving reality. And I circle true. I didn't circle false. I circled true.

(P): And it matches up.

(T): It matches up, right? (Rhetorical)

(P): Right.

(T): So, the one thing you said is that it matches up, that means that it's correlating, I think that's the word you used.

(P): Yeah correlating to reality.

(T): All right, that is a possibility. What is another possibility?

(P): That's a person's brain, we'll say, and that is how they are perceiving.

(T): That, what, every time they perceive something then it is correct. Is it?

(P): I mean if you're circling it. You're circling true and actuality and then it goes back to reality then I am going to assume yeah.

(T): You are going to assume. That assumption is the reason I did it. Again, you cannot know why I did it. You can't know why I would do it. It could be. I might have thought of that idea. What is another possibility if that is a person's brain perceiving reality, their actuality is true, is there a problem with that, from what we said so far?

(P): Well, I mean, if it is just an interpretation, it doesn't, I mean, they think it is true, it doesn't mean that it is actually true. Is what you are trying to say?

(T): No, not exactly that's not what I was trying to say (laughter), but it incorporates what I was saying. They don't think that it doesn't necessarily.

(P): You mean that it's not true?

(T): They don't think that.

(P): Right.

(T): *They think, because I perceive it/interpret that way, it is true.* People think that what they think is true. They don't think they maybe what they are thinking is not true. Like I thought when you saw that, you would see the shape of a nut. I am teaching you this, right? And I didn't think you might perceive it differently because I wasn't being conscious of that. I was being conscious of something else. It is very slippery.

(P): Yeah.

(T): So the idea of this is to teach the brain to become very rigorous. Even now when I am doing it, even though I have done this for many years, that my brain may not be as rigorous as it could have been, and it can get more rigorous. Now it doesn't always have to be that rigorous. You know, if you were watching, if you were listening, I don't know, you could be doing activities where it (thinking) doesn't have to be quite that rigorous.

(P): Like driving?

(T): Yeah, but you know again, you know you can say that and then you realize it is better to be rigorous about a lot of things.

(P): Right.

(T): If you're driving you might want to realize.

(P): You should be.

(T): I mean, I don't know about you but I do check myself frequently when driving. (Asking myself) Are you conscious of what is going on around you? Are you paying attention?

(P): I use that example a lot about driving because sometimes you drive the same route all the time that it becomes a habit. And so you have to go a different route and you're not consciously just being mindful, cause I've done that before. You end up going the same route even though you're supposed to be going someplace else.

(T): Yeah very common ... So the idea here is to be a little bit more rigorous in our thinking. Particularly if it is something, if it is a couple, coming to you as a therapist that they're learning, that we are not very rigorous in our thinking. Now we may be very rigorous sometimes and not at others. So one example that I give is that a physician may be very rigorous in his/her thinking when doing surgery ... gets out of surgery and then goes home and how s/he thinks when doing surgery might not be a bad idea to be thinking that rigorously when talking to his or her children or spouse. It does happen that people's brain under different circumstances work differently. We'll talk about that later.

All right, so we get to *the second step, which is determining whether our actuality (interpretation/construct) is either true or false. We want the couple to be aware of that as we go through this whole process.*
I just want to insert this now. Aristotle talked about the idea of defining terms. He made a statement about the importance of defining the meaning of a word. And, his admonishment in more words or less was, if you do not define a word, if it does not have a meaning, then there is no meaning at all. Therefore, we could not (verbally) communicate with others, because there is no meaning. Further, without the definition or meaning of terms or concepts, we would not be able to construct meaning or to understand or extrapolate our experiences in the conscious manner seemingly unique to human beings. Again, my *belief* is that Aristotle didn't just say that without a purpose, but that he was saying it for a reason. It is that he wanted us to understand his predecessors; Socrates and Plato talked about certain *concepts*. If you do not define the meaning of those concepts, then you do not understand what they (the concepts or the great thinkers) mean ... So, I thought that was a way of him saying that when you learn these concepts from people like Plato you need to understand what they mean. This is so we can understand how these concepts are interrelated (Conceptual Template) allowing us to understand the concepts our mind is using in a more intelligible way, in order to think and communicate more clearly, and so that we minimize using a word incorrectly, misinterpreting, misunderstanding and so on. We know this when we use a word incorrectly, as it sometimes changes the whole meaning. I'll give you an example of that.
Let's imagine that a woman came from a home in which they would say whatever they felt when upset or angry with another family member. Now, imagine a woman in this family married a man. That man came from a family that wouldn't say certain things; it was strictly forbidden. For example, a child would not ever say a "bad" word, particularly to a mother. I don't know about to a father, maybe not even then. But the other family would. Both families might scream and yell at each other, but the man's family would never use a word that could be interpreted as literally hurtful. The woman's family might say, "I hate you!" And ten minutes later it is all over, forgotten or forgiven. The husband's family would never say that. It would have been taken literally.
This imaginary couple comes to you for counseling, presenting when the wife would get very upset with the husband, like in your example about sex. Let's change your example. She wanted to have more sex, not less. Nevertheless, she would get very angry when she wanted to have sex and he didn't want to have sex with her. She would then say, "I hate you, I hate your guts."

He was so hurt by that because his family never said, "I hate you!" as their interpretation would be, literally, I hate you. He would then feel so dejected that he did not want to have sex with her for days, even weeks, which exacerbated the issue. How might you help them using the Conceptual Template?

By using the Conceptual Template, it would help them understand that when she said, "I hate you" she did not mean that she actually hated him. It meant that she felt rejected and unloved and therefore was very angry with him, which is a whole different interpretation or construct of the reality experienced. Having learned that and understanding how she actually felt, he became more understanding. She was able to respond by not using the word hate. He learned not to react with rejection but rather also with understanding, in that he knew she did not hate him when she got angry. Eventually being able to communicate through understanding the meaning of what was said or their behavior, this issue could to some extent be resolved at least to a degree that they could better communicate.

So, that is an imaginary example of understanding that words have a particular meaning. We want our clients to understand the definitions of these concepts so they can, for one, *understand how these concepts are interrelated, allowing them to form a construct of what the reality is and enable them to communicate with a better understanding.*

So, when we interpret something it could be either true or false; that is what you said. If something is true, what does that mean?

(P): That it correlates with reality. It correlates

(T): Right. I think we want it to be a stronger definition.

(P): Ok.

(T): Because something can correlate and not be true. Correlate is not the right word. The great thinkers actually went through this, questioning what the right word is. What might be another word?

(P): If something is true it matches up with what the reality is.

(T): That's pretty good. That is much better. It matches up with it. So if something matches.

(P): It is the same.

(T): That's good. Most of the great thinkers from Western civilization said, it *corresponds* with reality. But again something can correspond with reality in your mind and in reality not actually correspond exactly the way it is. "Matching." I never heard anybody say that, that is another good way to put it.

There was a man by the name of Yogananda and he said, truth corresponds *exactly* with reality, I think that is the word he used. But that idea of matching, or corresponding ... in science we see that all the time. People will think because something correlates that it is true and it may not be. It has to be exactly the way it is. So you want your clients to understand that is what truth means. And if something does not correspond exactly it might be partly true, I don't know, but if it were false then it would not correspond with reality. It would what? If your interpretation of something is false, then what's its relationship to reality?

(P): There is not, there is no relationship to reality. Right?

(T): Yeah.

(P): I mean there could be some relationship but it is not completely the same.

(T): Yeah. So just what I did here … I am sort of just talking with you. And when you work with a client (couple), it is not different. Even though this information is written down exactly (in the Instructional Manual) all the possible responses, probably not all of them (the most common or frequent) and therefore seems very rigorous and very exact, which it attempts to be when you are in a counseling relationship, you are two people talking with one another; you are trying to understand what is being communicated, just like this. And for people to understand this, you might have to switch gears in how you say something, depending upon the individual(s).

(P): And I think it is important like when you write it out like that it looks black and white, whether it is either true or false, right? And when people think about it they think it has to be 100% true or 100% false, but that is not true. You could be 99% true but there is still that 1% that is not true, and so it doesn't mean it is 100% reality. People think it is black or white a lot especially if they're coming to counseling, so making that clear to them that even though that 99% of what they feel think and know could be true, it doesn't mean that it is still reality.

(T): Ok, could you give an example of that?

(P): In relation to couples counseling?

(T): That would probably be good.

(P): Ok so let's say the wife feels she is doing all of the work at home. She takes the kids to school, she makes the meals, and she cleans up, because the husband works a lot. She knows that, but she feels that she has to take the brunt of the responsibility. And she does. You know she has all of this evidence that she is doing so much. But she is saying that her husband doesn't do anything at all to help So he comes home, he's tired, he works long hours, he eats, he doesn't help out, and so *in her mind* he doesn't do anything. But in reality, maybe he does the dishes once a week but she discounts that because it is not enough for her. She does the majority of the work.

Note to reader: In the example given by the practitioner, the issue thus far is in regard to what is considered fair/just.(T): So how she is expressing it, is not corresponding exactly … it is her interpretation. In a certain way it is true, that in general he doesn't do most things…

(P): Yeah, in general. But it is not 100% true that he's useless or doesn't do anything. She may use the words and those are like fighting or attacking words. Or she says washing dishes isn't a big deal. That doesn't count as helping. It is not validating what he actually does, but in her mind (actuality) it is still true that he doesn't do anything.

(T): So it is in her mind.

(P): Yeah.

(T): So when we think like that, I do not know if you know the word, but it is *in her mind* that washing the dishes is not a big thing; it could be *in his mind*, that it is a huge thing.

(P): Right.

(T): What do we call that? In reality that is a true statement, I can even prove that statement, I think it is self-evident, one person can hate washing the dishes, like oh my gosh I have to wash the dishes again. Someone else can just love it and they want to do the dishes all the time; they'll "fight" you to get to do the dishes. Do you know that or not?

(P): Yeah, it's possible.

(T): There are people who love to do the dishes. Or, clean the house. But if one person likes doing something and another one doesn't, what term could we use about that? That is being what? There is a term for that.

(P): A term for what?

(T): One person likes something and another person doesn't, it's really purely what?

(P): Subjective?

(T): Yes, subjective. That you may have gotten from way back. This is also where you may introduce it early on in therapy. If they don't know it, you introduce it. And you might even have a couple go home, look it up, think about it, and give examples of it. So at this point we want to say that our *actuality* would be what?

(P): Inaudible...

(T): Our actuality has to be what?

(P): At this point? (Laughter)

(T): Yeah, when we interpret something our actuality at this point has to be what?

(P): True or false

(T): Yes it has to be true or false. And now we are interpreting it, at that point initially anyway, it is what? You are interpreting it, so it could be true or false, so therefore, it has got to be what because initially it is what?

(P): Right or wrong?

(T): Well that is also true. But at that point you do not know whether it is right or wrong. Right? That is what you do, like I am doing it (getting the couple to figure out what is being said), so it is what at that point?

(P): Well it is not true or false it's just kind of like gathering information.

(T): Yes, it is kind of like gathering information. And so at that point you are gathering information. A lot of it is what?

(P): It is not being interpreted yet.

(T): No, it is being interpreted.

(P): You have information, and you're interpreting it

(T): Yeah, all of it, trying to figure out if it is true.

(P): You are experiencing it.

(T): Yes, you are experiencing, and it is either true or false, so what do you have to do when you are interpreting something and you are aware that it is either true or false, which is the idea, you want them to be aware, if you are aware consciously that your...

(P): You are analyzing it.

(T): You are analyzing it or you might what? Rather than making an assumption, you might what?

(P): Rather than making an assumption you might believe that that it is true.

(T): You could believe that is true. If you *believe* that it is true, you are being what?

(P): You are being biased.

(T): You are being biased. You are being, what else?

(P): *Subjective?*

(T): Subjective, but that is what people do. They react. Sensory information comes in, it automatically goes to their putting it together in some form through their interpretation, and they think it is true. Generally they do not go beyond that. If you are more scientific, which is rigorous, you might do what with regard to what you think is true?

(P): You'll kind of take a step back and kind of look at it and reexamine the information.

(T): Yeah you might do that. So, in the Conceptual Template, there are a lot of ways to say this, it is not just the Steps, but the third step you would question it. You say, "Step back." So prior to stepping back whatever a person thinks at this point is subjective, and it is important to be aware of that, that is just their initial understanding of something. When they do this, if you are questioning then, they are being what?

(P): *Objective.*

(T): Very good! And so now, since you question (Step 3), you're moving into stepping back, which, is how sometimes, people talk about what objective thinking is. So it is a good thing to have the couple, *at this juncture, to clearly differentiate or to understand the difference between subjectivity and objectivity or subjective and objective thinking.* How are you doing?

(P): Good!

(T): So far that makes a lot of sense. Right?

(P): Yeah

(T): So what we normally do ... I am not quite sure why this happens, but it is commonplace, people think that whatever they think is true. And it is lickety-split.

(P): Yeah well our brain needs to do that because it is the simplest way to think.

(T): Right, and why might that be important?

(P): Because otherwise we would be overloaded with information, things would be too complicated to figure things out. It tries to make connections the quick and simplest way it can. But it doesn't mean it is right.

(T): So when we are conscious of that, like what you are saying, we might then realize what? When we think this is what happens, because otherwise we would be overloaded, but what we are communicating about with our partner is really important, because you're upset, I am upset, or what have you, and therefore rather than just overloading, we are going to do what?

(P): We're going to take a step back and to kind of take it in first, and really examine what we are experiencing, through our perceptions. Like if we are angry, realizing where that anger is coming from and not reacting right away. Make sure that we are angry for the right reasons and not just because we misinterpret what is going on.

(T): Yes, good, exactly. Can you think of any other reason why our brain might do that?

(P): What, simplify things?

(T): Yes.

(P): Just because it is easier.

(T): People will answer that question in different ways. There can be different ways that reactive behavior can be interpreted. But that is what our brain does. And so we need to slow it down in important circumstances and reflect on how we choose to act. Is this the way I responded, was that really the best way to respond? It could be fifteen, twenty minutes later and you are with your spouse and you say "Look, I gave you the answer," like a "typical" male, that is what women often say, or I have heard women in couple counseling express that often men don't listen, men want to fix it all the time. If a women says something and he is ready to fix it and the women is upset because he didn't let her express what she was feeling, and that was all that she needed, she doesn't need a man to tell her how to think, which I think is part of that too. Certainly that idea, that a male thinking that he can think better than the female, and the woman being somewhat subjugated to the male throughout history.

(P): People are so stuck with what they're feeling that it is hard for them to take a step back from their feelings and not react and really listen to what the other person has to say.

(T): That is the way our brain works. Part of this reactive response has to do with the limbic system. That is the old part of the brain. This is something you can explain to couples also. I think it is good for people to learn meditation in order for the relaxation response to kick in.

I questioned meditation, when I first learned it in my early 20s, all the way to the time when Guru Maharishi Yogi introduced Western Culture to Transcendental Meditation. I learned different types. I use to think people were goofy when I use to work going door-to-door selling the Great Books of the Western World, sometimes in the student dorms, and I would see students meditating, sometimes in their closet. I would think, what is wrong with everybody here? After a while I learned there was empirical research that found that mediation could cause the "relaxation response" to occur; it is a physiological response emanating from the limbic system. When there is a fight or flight response, mediation can calm it down. The relaxation response might not appear to be a big deal, but it is because it is an autonomic response of our nervous system, it respond automatically. So mediation is a method by which we can control our autonomic nervous system. It is very nice to know how to do that, for example if heart rate is all of a sudden increasing to a high level because of some situation and you don't want that to happen, you can meditate and slow it down. You can save your life with it. It is very important for couples, for people in general, in my opinion, today, I don't think it is opinion, it is based upon more than opinion, the research indicates it has a real objective value. I could also give other reasons, but nevertheless I really questioned its actual value..

(P): You don't even have to go as deep as mediation. Just deep breathing will calm them.

(T): Yeah, sure. You can do that too. The reason I think meditation can be important is because you might use it later on for something of real value that people might not realize at the time ... It might be particular to the individual. For example, even when I started writing this book a few years ago, although I had meditated on a regular basis, I didn't meditate specifically right before I started writing each day. But one day I came into my office and started meditating just to relax a little bit. Then I started writing and I realized things were a lot easier or clearer. Now I meditate before I write because everything is clearer; I am not anxious, and am more receptive.

Ok, so we are talking about being reflective, not reacting, but our brain normally reacts in circumstances that are perceived by the brain to be threatening, This is because the limbic system does not think, it is the old part of the brain which reacts to perceived danger for survival. Adrenalin increases, the heart rate increases, blood vessels dilate, blood carrying nutrients is pumped more quickly to the muscles, and the animal or person has increased strength to fight or flee. But this response is for survival, and so what we can do when the fight or flight response is not necessary, is to stop, think, and to question our response or action or choice in order to be more objective about our own subjectivity and choice of how we respond. Therefore, *the one thing you want to be aware of, maybe the conclusion to all this, is that it is critically important for a person to be aware, to be objective of or about their own subjectivity as much as they are aware of the subjectivity of others and what that is.* And, I think you said to me the other day ... you said to me that the people you work with, their conflict is about what? Well I will remind you, and if I am wrong you can say I never said that.

(P): Ok.

(T): Which may or may not be true. It may or may not correspond to reality. You said most people's ... issues are, they're subjective. Do you remember saying that?

(P): No. (Laughter)

(T): Wow! Isn't that interesting? And then I said, could you give me an example? You don't remember that?

(P): Is that when I was talking about the...

(T): No ... You just said that most couple's conflict is subjective, and I said that it would be great if you could give some examples.

(P): Oh, ok.

(T): ...Do you remember that or not?

(P): Yes.

(T): Ok, so sometimes what is not so important to you, in my mind it is very important. Can you see the value of understanding that generally people are subjective and then you being objective about their subjectivity?

(P): Yeah.

(T): If we learn anything about this today, *that's a critical point for a couple to learn it is, to become more objective not only about their own subjectivity, most importantly, and then also aware of the subjectivity of another or others.* And because of that, we need to question our interpretation. As I mentioned earlier, Freud said, the greatest cathexis is to the self, which I think meant, our ego always thinks we are right. OK, are we done?

(P): Yes, we're done.

(T): See, now my interpretation of your movement was, we're done.

(P): Yeah, so that part was good. Because I totally forgot about that part, the subjective thinking, I mean being objective about our own subjectivity. That's really important.

(T): That's very important. Good. So, it's a good review so far.

(P): Yeah, it has been a good review.

SESSION 2: PART 2 REVIEW OF FIRST SESSION. THE ESSENTIAL CONCEPT OF
KNOWLEDGE

(T): Do you want to try to recall what we did last time in the first part of the CT? You could talk about what you learned.

(P): I forgot how far we got.

(T): Ok, well I looked back at the transcript (Laughter). It was a little hard to figure out.

(P): It's hard to figure out?

(T): Well, sometimes. And also the other thing that I think which is important for someone who is learning this is, I do jump back and forth a little bit, and I don't think it's harmful, of course that might be a rationalization, to jump back and forth, because I believe it makes a person have to think, "Where were we?" Just like what you are doing right now. I even had to go back. But everything relates to one thing, and what we are always trying to figure out, and I will just sort of guide this, and that is what a person should do when teaching this. We're always trying to do or determine what? Basically, we are always trying to determine what as human beings?

(P): Reality.

(T): Yeah, we are trying to figure out reality. We need to figure out reality because? Why is that important?

(P): To survive.

(T): Yes, to survive. And beyond the surviving, because we are not just surviving, what else?

(P): To be happy.

(T): To be happy, right. I am not sure if animals do that but we certainly do. So this is sort of a review, we (Humans) are always trying to understand reality. When you are working with somebody, and I am doing this so practitioners as well as others who have an interest can learn this. The first thing you want them to understand is, the meaning of the term reality. Right? You defined the term reality as being what?

(P): Things that are real, and things that are objective, that we all can agree upon, that reality is what is.

(T): "Reality is what is," is a good way to put it. We then interpret it. An *interpretation of reality* is actually *a construct of reality*. That is our *actuality*, *a construct of reality* when we do what you are talking about. But now that we have formed that construct, and you are saying that is reality, another way to say that is really human beings have a construct of reality. So really what you are saying is, we're trying to figure out what is? What is the construct that we are trying to figure out? What is, not just realty, but in our mind's, what is what, blank or blank might be a way to put it. It is what I ask couples.

(P): True or false.

(T): Yeah, we're trying to figure out *what is true or false*. But even when you are working with a couple, or anybody, you want them to understand that *reality just is that which exists, and we're not saying what it is, so you are never imposing on a person what they should or shouldn't think*. My *personal opinion* of that is anybody can be wrong. Remember that little nut we drew, the way people think means that they *believe that what they think is true*.

For example, the other night I was with Steve (A friend). We are driving into a parking lot at night, and the pavement was wet and I said, "Oh it must have rained here." And he said, something to the effect of "You think it rained here? Or, could it be something else?" And I said, "Well it could have been something else." He said, "It is the sprinkler system." So, apparently, he must have seen the sprinkler system. I didn't see that. But he was making a point, and in his mind he is "always" thinking well it could be true or it may not be true. We can be absolutely sure in our mind that something is true, and it just is not. And, so we always need to, and that is *the second point, once we have in our mind that something is true, we can immediately think, it could be false*, as sure as I am, it could be false. Or as you put it last time, *it may be 99% true but there might be something we are not seeing in it*. All right, so that is *the first and second step, that we are determining (or asking ourselves) "What is the reality?" It is the second step or our interpretation or construct of reality that we then can we keep in abeyance; it is either true or false. In the third step we do what? Do you remember what that is?*

(P): You find evidence.

(T): We might do that, but we would first, yeah, we would have to *question* it, and then we would look for evidence. So your earlier point that when we stand back we are being sort of what about our thinking? *If we are standing back like you said, we are really being what now?*

(P): Objective.

(T): Objective, right. And so in the second step when we are aware of our interpretation or as indicated on the CT, actuality being either true or false, but it cannot be both true and false at the same time. Even if we think our interpretation or actuality is true, it is subjective at that point. So as you say, we attempt to get evidence, and that is being objective.

... *at that point* where it could be true or false, when the person/couple could step into that subjectivity by taking a position or stance and stay there, *is to bring up the idea of getting them to define what subjectivity is, and to distinguish that from objectivity*. So we are trying to be objective throughout this process, and we are aware that there is always going to be a certain level of subjectivity no matter how objective we are.

The third step is questioning, seeking evidence, or even more rigorously seeking evidence to prove ourselves to be incorrect (Null hypothesis); we are doing all of this, questioning, seeking evidence and so on in order to determine whether or not what we are thinking is either true or false. And, we may be doing that with regard to what somebody else is saying or interpreting, because they also have a kind of subjectivity, even if they have objectivity. All right, *so you start looking for evidence and you are doing that because at this point you really don't, what/blank, whether your thinking is true or false?* This is the next question I ask couples.

(P): You *don't know.*

(T): You *do not know,* right. So that is the forth step, it is *knowledge,* you have to determine whether or not you *know, i.e. whether something is true or false.* And in the instance I gave you, with Steve, did I *know?*

(P): Right.

(T): So you can *know* something, you can be *not sure* of something, and you can also *not know something.* But a person has to determine *whether they know, do not know or are not sure.* And the only way we really *know* that what we are thinking is true, which means it corresponds *exactly* (Yogonanda) to reality, that's the word I checked on that, "exactly" to reality, is to have what? You would have to be able to what? You talked about evidence? Again this is what I would ask a couple in couple counseling.

(P): You would have to have *proof.*

(T): Yes you would have to have *proof,* in a single word, that's what it is. And, you would have to look at that *proof objectively* to determine that it has validity too. Because people will say that something is proven, like in a courtroom. I sometimes watch these shows on television to see how people think, and ... it is entertaining, maybe not entertaining in a way, but you wonder, how can they come to that conclusion; they just don't know. It is obvious they don't know, but because the community.as an example, wants a conviction, they may be influenced to convict somebody and the individual might go to jail for life. And, that has really happened over and over and over. We have proof of that, that juries make mistakes. People are convicted for heinous crimes that they are not guilty of and may serve a life term or be put to death. This is how serious this can be. In our own lives, we also *need to know* like that. So, being aware of our own *actuality (our interpretation/construct)* our own subjectivity, being aware of another person's actuality and their subjectivity, we often don't know what that is. So we need to determine that sometimes, or we move forward and we find out. But, *the only way we know is that we have objective proof. Therefore truth is an exact correspondence between thought and reality. That which contradicts reality is false. And knowledge is a proven correspondence between thought, and reality. Without proof one does not know or is not sure.*

(P): Right.

(T): So I will give you an example. Yesterday when I was trying to communicate with you with regard to meeting here today, Sunday ... I really sort of noticed how I didn't know how you thought. I didn't want to be imposing on you. I was thinking, or in my mind (My actuality, interpretation, or subjective construct), I thought, oh it is Sunday, that might not be a good day for her; she wants to be home with her family. I forgot you do therapy sometimes in the morning on Sunday. But for me Sunday is, like football (Laughter). And, I had to go over or question my own *subjectivity by being more objective.* If you are on vacation for a couple of weeks, I need to be working on this transcript when you are gone.

(P): Yeah.

(T): But I just went ahead, and I gave you an option, would Monday be better, and then you told me you were coming in anyway maybe that would be good on Sunday. So then I *knew,* I thought oh that's right, my subjectivity that I might be imposing on you was really strong, I almost used the words, "I hope I am not imposing on you." But I did *not know* that I was, so I didn't use the term. But objectively it was not an imposition necessarily, if you stayed here for another hour. Ok, so that is the first part.

So now we understand that all we are trying to figure out is the reality, all the way through this whole thing (CT). It gets more complicated – the second half. *Knowledge is a proven correspondence between our thought and reality.* So whatever we think is true, *if we can prove that it is true, than we have knowledge.*

Again, I just want to say that *knowledge is a process,* and so knowledge is not just some piece, stuck, fixed, nothing on the edges of it; we always want to keep our mind's open, but we can have sort of fixed knowledge. For example, when the astronauts were coming back, when they were landing on the moon, they let's take had to be *exactly right.* Any slight deviation could have been the end of their lives. So there is exact correspondence between what we think and reality. Mathematics does that. Some people *believe* mathematics is the only reality because of that (exactness). But however we cut it, our mind's, you know, as long as we are aware, *our mind has to be open to possibilities, not getting absolutistic, not becoming dogmatic, but also not becoming so loose in our thinking that we say well there is no way to really determine what is true.* Many people do think like that, not maybe in every area of their life, but in some area. And, the next area we are going into, that's where they do it in a way that in my opinion can be very harmful. I use the word opinion, so again when you do this with somebody, you might just use a word, and again you have to have the whole conceptual idea in your mind of what we are doing. Note: *We are identifying how our mind by its very nature, uses specific and essential concepts and their interrelationships to understand (have knowledge) of reality in order to then make choices that are rational and objectively of value in order to survive, thrive, and to experience value in our existence or to be, to some extent, content and happy.*

I didn't use the word opinion. I may not have used that for a while, you may have used it later, I may have forgotten it, gone back to it, but I just used it, so now I will use it, in the first part of this paradigm we can have knowledge, but you may also think, I am not sure that it is true, or I don't know that it is true, then that would not constitute knowledge, that would constitute what?

(P): Just information.

(T): Just information, or an (blank)? If you don't know it, you may what, it's your (blank)?

(P): Your belief.

(T): Your belief. You didn't use the word opinion. So that's good. Is a belief and an opinion similar or the same?

(P): I think it is similar.

(T): Yeah it is certainly similar. Again *you want the couple to understand that there is a difference between an opinion or a belief and knowledge.* That is important because an opinion or belief is different from knowledge. An opinion or belief differs from knowledge in that an opinion or belief is thinking or interpreting some issue as being true but there is no <u>Blank</u>.

(P): Proof.

(T): Good, or objective proof, and *therefore it is subject to doubt.* Therefore knowledge is <u>Blank</u> and an opinion or belief is <u>Blank</u>?

(P): Subjective and one is objective

(T): Which is which?

(P): An opinion, or what you believe is subjective.

(T): Good. So when I had that comment made to me (by Steve), I don't know if the word belief was used or not, but that was the idea, that was probably said more in jest, but what is said in jest, might "jest" (just) be the truth. (Steve was really asking) Are you thinking? Are you being objective? I know what that is, when we do that, it is just sort of jostling a little bit, just to be funny. But it is serious ... I don't think he thinks that I think that way. I hope he doesn't (Laughter) given, after I did all this work for so many years. But it can happen. I've done it even if I understand this 100%. I catch myself thinking you don't know that. You don't have sufficient evidence for that. So we want the client(s) to understand that in being objective, we have to have knowledge, or objective proof, that we have objective evidence, that what we think is true, that it actually a corresponds exactly to the reality. Just like going out into outer space, there are things like that. If you are giving medication to somebody, it's got to be, maybe, exact. Off a little bit, it could have serious consequences, kill them. I think in even being a good therapist you have to be exact, and you have to be precise. It doesn't mean all the time, but if you are working with couples you need to know exactly what you are doing. I don't think this is oh just let's see how we talk about this and how we go back and forth subjectively. And I think sometimes that can be the case that the practitioner/person is not recognizing the subjectivity of what is going on and they are not going to be helping the person or couple. Hopefully most psychologists are fairly objective. The only way to know that would be to study that (Laughter). All right, we'll go to the second half now (of the CT).

All right, so *the first half of this CT is to understand (have knowledge of) what the reality is and differentiate it from our interpretation, belief or opinion of what* it is. Once we understand what the reality is, the next thing is, we are trying to understand reality in order, for what (purpose)? Why would anyone want to understand reality, not just for theoretical reasons, that might be one reason, out of curiosity, but what is the other reason that we would need to understand reality?

(P): Is it what I said earlier, in order to be happy?

(T): Yeah, that's true, so in order to survive or to be happy. So once we have an understanding of the reality that we are experiencing, what is the purpose, it might be to be happy or to survive but now it is going to do what for us?

(P): So you make better decisions?

(T): *So we can make better decisions, exactly, right. So it is really guiding our decisions making or guiding our actions. Give me an example of something where you made a decision lately. (Note: Guiding practitioner/client toward understanding the concept of value and its purpose).*

(P): I made a decision to *take* a trip to Japan for the second time this year.

(T): All right twice this year. That's very nice. And you made that decision because?

(P): So, Initially I didn't want to go because I felt like it would cost too much; we were just there, the kids would miss school. So I was really against it. However, I thought about the *value* of family time and if we could afford to go and having experiences then we should just go because we don't know when we can do that again, together, all of us.

(T): You used the word *value*.

(NOTE: When client(s) use an essential concept it is important to point out that it is a natural aspect of cognition. In this way, they will realize it is natural or part of the nature of human reasoning; you are just helping them to realize it, as well as the value of being mindful of this natural process.)

I don't know if that is the way you normally speak or not. You implied another thing, that we both really wanted to go, and we thought it would really be good for the kids and they wanted to go and you would be using a term like *want*. Whether it would be worthwhile for the family, *all of those terms could be coalesced into one term* which would be what you are *valuing*. You just happened to use the word *value*. *So when you are working with a couple, or anybody, somehow you want to bring that out, that it is natural, they do it all the time* they just aren't aware of it. You can give them an example, which illustrates that if you have awareness or consciousness of how something works you can improve what you are doing, in this instance improving reasoning. If a child observes and is taught by a parent how to build a canoe they will learn how to do that with the reasoning necessary to more readily build a canoe when they are older). Now I just did it in a particular way, that's a little subjective. I just sort of know where I am going, and know what I want to do. So for you, it is the same thing. You want the person to recognize in the first part (of the CT) it is just to understand (what is meant by the word) *reality*. Because if you don't understand the reality or what is meant by the term reality, the likelihood that you are going to choose what you are going to do in a way that it somehow moves toward or is consonant with the reality is less likely, if not unlikely. So, *value* is the next concept, and you want them to understand that essential concept used in the conceptual process. So if we use the word value and again with each step you take we want the individuals to understand the meaning of the term. *Humans need to understand the meaning of words for what reason?* We talked about this last time.

(P): *So that we can all agree on what all of it means (Laughter) can have the same understanding.*

(T): Yes, that's what it is all about. And in our own brain that it is the same understanding. (Note: this is the basis of human communication.) So that is another point I brought up before, but I am bringing it up again. You say it really well. A lot of people don't say that, so that we have a sort of universal language. That is the problem, people do not necessarily understand the other persons meaning. They don't understand the reality (or the other's actuality). Conflict arises and then they are going off in different directions, they are not pinning it down, that this is the reality, we both agree this is the reality. Now that we *know* that (the next question/concern we have is) now what do we *value*? If we want to go in this direction, *we need to identify that and what value means*. And it just means something that is worthwhile or what we want. But if we think about values, then *the next thing to do is ask a couple to separately list what each of them values.*

Could I ask you to just do that for a minute, to write that down?

(P): You want me to write it down on the board?

(T): Yeah, that would make it real easy.

(P): Family
Health

Weight lifting

My free time, which I don't have much of (Laughter)

Work

Friends

Relationships, I think that would be the same

Our ability to live comfortable, like living comfortably, we make money so we

can live comfortably and to provide for our kids, to not have to worry so much

Air conditioning

My vacuum, top of the line vacuum

(T): Try a couple more

(P): Physical strength

A good mother, for sure

Being a strong women for my daughters, a role model

(T): Just put another one up there.

(**Note**: Practitioners can also rephrase and ask clients, particularly if they have difficulty identifying what they value, *"What would you not want to be denied?"*)

(P): My house.(T): Usually making a list of values is a take home assignment. The practitioner is encouraged to get as an extensive list as possible. Then *the couple is asked to separate their list of values into two categories.*

The first category is: *"Those things that you value, that all rational people value, even if they are not aware of it." And to separate that out from:*

"Those things you value, that other rational people may also value, but not necessarily all rational people would value."

(P): Ok.

(T): So for example, (using her list) which category would family fit into? Do all rational people value family?

(P): Yes.

(T): Yeah, I would think so.

(P): Yeah, I would think so.

(T): How about health? Do all rational …

(P): Yes

(T): Do all rational people value weightlifting?

(P): No.

(T): No, so that is a different category. That is other rational people might value but not all rational people would value.

(T): Free time. Do all rational people value free time?

(P): I think so.

(T): Yeah, maybe. It could go one-way or another. There might be some people who really

(P): Like keeping busy and

(T): Yeah, and really don't have a need for it. But if we change that word to freedom to choose what you do with your time, would all rational people value that?

(P): Yes.

(T): So we could separate that and you could do that with a couple too, to separate that out. Work, do all rational people value work?

(P): Maybe not, yeah rational people.

(T): People do just what you did. They'll think some people don't like to have to work at all, but they value work whether or not they like their work, even if unaware that they do. If you work in a place where we don't have the kind of formalized kind of working we have in this culture or other Western cultures or Eastern cultures, somebody living in the Bolivian rainforest for example, in order for them to get food, by definition, even by what that means in physics, they have to work. They have to climb a tree to get a snake or fruit ... And so we all, all rational people value work because if we didn't work.

(P): We wouldn't get what we want or need.

(T): Need, right. Ok, good.

(T): Friends, do all rational people value friends?

(P): Yeah, I think so...

(T): Yeah, I don't know.

(P): Yeah, I don't know. It could go either way.

(T): *It could go either way. And it doesn't have to be exact here. But we want the person (couple) to get the idea of what we are doing here.*

(P): Right.

(T): What about relationships? Do all people value relationships?

(P): I think so.

(T): Yeah, I think so. No matter what it could be, certainly a child and its mother. If a child doesn't have a relationship with its mother during infancy, what I mean by that, an intimate relationship with its mother, that could be, that is generally pretty harmful. We already know that.

(T): To live comfortably. Do all...

(P): Yeah.

(T): Yeah.

(P): Whatever that means to them.

(T): Yeah whatever that means to them. A lot of people don't think of that. When they meet somebody, they don't think can I live comfortably with this individual. I see a lot, and your shaking your head like you see a lot too.

(P): Right.

(T): People can get into a relationship with somebody who's not going to put forth effort in providing, at least, equally, in some form, and it puts a lot of strain in the relationship because they can't afford the basic necessities. And you know the saying "Love conquers all," but when that kind of thing is happening unless you are working together in concert, to make a comfortable living, that could become very traumatic. It is very different than two people being together and both people working very hard and maybe they are not comfortable for a number of years, in the sense of things you are talking about, like being able to get a Rainbow vacuum, (Laughter), but if that is what they are working toward together to have a comfortable life, it is "working" together is important. That has what kind of value that they're both working together to be comfortable together? That has what kind of value to them?

(P): What do you mean?

(T): We will come back to that. Ok, the value you listed of being strong, let's do that one.

(P): Being strong? Not everyone.

(T): Do all rational people whether they are aware of it or not value being strong?

(P): No, I mean strong as in like weightlifting strong. Strong as in healthy strong, I think yeah.

(T): Yeah, good. So, you separated that out.

(P): Uh huh.

(T): Even physically strong is important. If your legs are not physically strong when you get older, or your arms aren't, you can't do things. I mean you *need* physical strength. Weight lifting is a little different That is where you are going beyond normal strength, particularly in a culture here where people are not working all the time like they might in some cultures where they get strong because they are physically having to do many things.

So, next on your list, what about being a good mother? Is that something that all rational women...

(P): I think so.

(T): And that is difficult to really figure out by the way.

(P): What?

(T): What being a good mother is.

(P): Right.

(T): Like a mother might think "I have to be very strict". Another mother might think I need to be giving a lot of freedom. And how do you figure that all out. Again, that is the kind of objectivity that a person might want to consider. How do I know what that is?

(P): Right, just defining the word good...

(T): Exactly, very good … Being a good role model for your children … Do you think all rational women would value that?

(P): I think so.

(T): How about a house? (Laughter) Do all rational women value a house?

(P): Yes, a house, but I think some would want a bigger house than others.

(T): If I were to use a different term like shelter, would that be different than a house?

(P): Yes.

(T): So do all rational people value a shelter?

(P): Maybe I should have put a home.

(T): A home that would be different.

(P): Right.

(T): So we might want to distinguish that, just for this purpose. *So what we have really done here is we have divided these values into two categories. I just didn't say what those categories were. Can you figure out what these categories are?*

(P): Objective or subjective.

(T): Very good. So *we want people to become aware of what they are valuing, as being either objectively or subjectively of value.* And, I think it is also important to explain that no matter how a person defines objectivity, it might be sort of standing back from things; many people say it that way. But an *objectively derived,* I think the word *derived is a good term, or based value means, it's based in reality.* You need shelter, whether it's a cave, or you build a shelter, it is where you live. A home is a wonderful thing to have, everybody might like it, or want it, but it is not objectively based in reality, a shelter is. *A subjectively derived value or subjectivity is basing it upon our actuality* or how we interpret those things around us. They're not a need, *so a good distinction to be made also, is a distinction between a want and a need. A want would be what kind of value?*

(P): A subjective…

(T): Correct. And obviously an objective value would be a need, even a metaphysical need. And you might want to define a metaphysical need. Do you know what a metaphysical, …no? Most people don't. Metaphysical is beyond the physical such as freedom. It's not a physical need, but it's a metaphysical need. …So metaphysical, there are a metaphysical objective things as well, like freedom, is a metaphysical need, more abstract not concrete. Ok, so *we want to differentiate or have couples differentiate objectively derived from subjectively derived values and understanding where each of them come from, because when you make a decision you might want to be aware of which is which.*

Then the next step is-… when we make a decision, you want to be aware of what you value so that you can make decisions; decisions are going to guide our actions. This is another thing you want them (a couple) to understand about what they are valuing. This is a conscious-awareness. Some people have this consciousness, without thinking of these concepts per se, but they are just very conscious like that. I think you're like that, pretty much. That is how I interpret you. Some people are less conscious-... the most conscious people are, not many. This one man who taught me a lot of things, he was 94 years old, living in the Himalayas, 40 years of silence. People thought he was a special kind of person. I think he really was a very special kind of person, certainly very intelligent, very conscious, and very rational and intuitive. He was the man who read my dissertation in one evening or overnight and talked to me about it in the morning. He said, "Change this one word." And that word was interpretation, second step, I don't know what word I had, I think I had perception. He said "Change it to "actuality." That had to do with a man, a book that was written about actuality ...a construct of reality (Krishnamurti). Nevertheless when we are making a decision we're either going to make a decision that something is an objectively derived value or it is something that is a subjectively derived value; that is the most common one.

(P): My friend went to the doctor recently, even though she has been working out for a while, she hasn't lost weight. Her doctor told her she had to lose 40 pounds.... That's a lot. So, this weekend was the County Fair. She enjoys eating. Even though we got her to start logging down her weight, or the things that she eats, and she is supposed to lose 40 pounds and to work on it, we went to the fair and she still ate a ton of food.

(T): Yeah, she can think of that a lot of ways, but if she was thinking about what is objectively of value and what is subjectively of value she would have chosen maybe to eat differently than she did. And that is a good example.

(P): Objectively she needs to lose the weight and eat healthy but subjectively she really likes county fair food.

(T): So that's what happens. The other possibility you can have other than an objective and subjective values coming into conflict, which we have been discussing is? What other values can come into conflict?

(P): Subjective vs. subjective.

(T): Yeah,

(P): Right, cotton candy,

(T): Yummy.

(P): Or a pronto pop, (Laughter)

(T): A what?

(P): A pronto pop.

(T): What is that?

(P): It is a specialty here. It is like a corn dog.

(T): All right, nevertheless, so when a subjective value and another sub-jective value come into conflict, how do you decide which one to use?

(P): I don't know. In the moment which I mean whichever one you feel like, because neither one has a greater value other than subjective preference.

(T): I think you said to me, if I recall, that the most common experience in therapy with couples or the issues they had was that they were what kind of problems? Do you remember?

(P): No.

(T): Subjective.

(P): Oh right.

(T): Do you remember that now?

(P): Yeah, yeah!

(T): Yeah, that's what it is. People get into these arguments, they fight; they don't talk to each other. It is often subjective. Even the example you gave which had to do with sex. Somebody wants to have sex more often than the other. It is purely subjective. There is objectivity in terms of maybe a certain level of need in the human body but it can vary based upon circumstances in life. So even if it has a certain level of subjectivity or a certain level of objectivity both people need to get objective about their subjectivity and even their objectivity. So two subjective values can create a conflict but it is fairly arbitrary; it is important to know that. So we can have an objective and subjective value, a subjective and subjective value comes into conflict, and what is the other one we can have?

(P): Objective and objective.

(T): Yes we can have an objective and objective, and this one is probably the most difficult. So what do you do when you have two objective values coming into conflict?

(P): I have an example.

(T): Great!

(P): So the husband has a really good job, but he works six days a week, for ten hours a day, hardly home, but he is making good money, he's providing for the family. So the family is comfortable. And then the wife who values their time together and wants him to be home more often although she understands they need this job because objectively it pays for the bills and to live comfortably. She also wants him home to spend time with the family. So the husband feels like he is being criticized for not spending enough time at home but he can't help it because he is a general manager of a business and it is an important job. And then the wife, who also works, but wants him to be home and present with the family.

(T) & (P): simultaneously say, "They're both objective."

(T): Yes they are both objective, but he has a responsibility even to main-tain that position, or for that business to be successful. So that is the most difficult obviously, right? And so we want to get people to the point that they can figure that one out. That can be figured out.

(P): Can it?

(T): Yes, it can be. At the 6th stage of (moral) development that one would be most readily resolvable, maybe at the 5th stage, but not so easily. So again the idea in all of this is to facilitate development to the highest stage we can get people. Certainly beyond Stage 4, hopefully because at Stage 5 there are certain things that go on that are extremely important that Stage 4 doesn't quite understand.

(**Note**: *The word right or rights, specifically moral right is omitted during this explanation so that the practitioners can discover this for themselves rather than being didactically told).*

(P): So when you are talking about the stages you are talking about stages of

(T): Moral development.

(P): Ok, so then do we talk about that with our clients?

(T): That is a really good question. Yeah, I think it is ok. You can tell people earlier on in the counseling process, or what have you, about stages of moral development. I usually do at some point, again early on, perhaps within the first three or four sessions.

(P): Right they're "gonna" talk about this and reference the stages someplace and you have to present that.

(T): Yeah. So again you are giving another good example. I'm glad you are doing it. I mean we're trying to do this in a way that is very concise. Normally, learning this takes, the research showed it took approximately 52 hours at one time. I cut it in half by giving homework assignments. But we are trying to do this in several sessions. But again, you brought up a couple of things that are critically important. And, you know when we finish you might have some questions and that might help. But yes, that is something (Stages) we would ordinarily introduce. Again it is having a real understanding of all this so you just know how to do it, one way or the other, even if it's at the end of the whole thing and you say, "one thing I would like to bring up by the way," and you go right back to it. It's getting to understand. Does this person (couple) have a grasp of what this all means? What stage are they really at? You know a person can sound like they are at Stage 5. That's not uncommon, which has to with "rights." Like somebody could say, well, they have a "right" to that and now the person that the therapist is thinking, oh, they must be Stage 5. But, that might just be a content response. They don't really understand what a right is. Like a kid can say, a parent says you are not going to use this today because you did this or that, they (child) say "I have a "right" to it; it is mine."

(P): Yeah, I remember I was thinking in elementary school and I think I got in trouble for something, and I said, "Well we are in America, it's my freedom, or I have the "right" to whatever (Laughter), and that didn't go well (Laughter).

(T): I am sure it didn't. Right, exactly. And you may have really had a right, but even if you have a right, you can have two rights come into conflict (objectively derived vs. objectively derived value).

(P): Yes.

(T): And then you have to figure out which one, they're both objective, so when you have two objective values come into conflict like that, how do you figure out which one is just? The one that is what?

(P): The one that, how do I know which one is fair or just? Well my parents say...

(T): Yeah, well it might be that, it might just be the authority, right? (Laughter)

But whenever we are trying to figure out, if we are trying to figure out which is an objective or subjective, you said an objective value supersedes a subjective value.

(P): Yeah.

(T): Because, why?

(P): Because everyone can agree on that.

(T): Yeah, that's one reason. And, it's more important.

(P): Right.

(T): Two subjective values, it's arbitrary. An objective and another objective you have, you can have two rights come into conflict.

(P): Right.

(T): That is usually the conflict at Stage 6. So you would have to be able to figure out, at least in terms of Stage 5, what? You have two objective values and you have to choose one. You choose the one that is what?

(P): Less harmful.

(T): Less harmful. (Acknowledging)

(P): That is more important.

(T): More important, and then if you learn Stage 6 which might be something we do or talk about, it might be worthwhile. Then there is a method to do this. And that is what is behind all of this. But when you have two rights come into conflict, now, but you can have a lot of subjective vs. subjective.

(P): Right.

(T): That is what you get most of the time.

(P): Yeah.

(T): Ok, so now we understand values. (To be continued)

SESSION 3: PRACTITIONER'S AND AUTHOR'S REVIEW. MORAL STAGES CLINICALLY EXPLORED MORAL DILEMMA SUGGESTED TO CLINICALLY MEASURE PRE AND POST CONVENTIONAL MORAL STAGE DEVELOPMENT AND FOR EVALUATING MORAL RELATIVISM

(T): Why don't we start today with a review. Start from the beginning of the Conceptual Template in your mind, all the way through values.

(P): Ok.

(T): Just so I have an understanding of what you understand, that is, your actuality.

(P): (Laughter) Ok, all right so, first you want to present to the client this template right? And the reason for it is so that they can understand their own thinking better. Then we introduce the concept of reality and we ask them "What does the term 'reality' mean?" "What do we mean by reality?" Ultimately the answer that we want (what we want them to understand) is reality is what it is. Then we introduce the concept of actuality, which is their perception of reality. And then we ask them "How do you know that their actuality matches reality?" Sometimes they say, well it does because when I think it is true, or real, kinda like that. (If the concept true were to be brought up spontaneously by the client, as would be the case with any essential concept in the CT, the practitioner then would have the client(s)/couple operationally define its meaning as well as how it relates to the concept being discussed). So then we try to get them to understand that in order to *know* if your actuality matches up with reality is you have to, kinda like a scientific experiment, you have to find proof. So you can either know, when you have proof, then you will know it matches reality, or you don't know because you haven't done your detective work. You know, don't know, or you are unsure. Those are the possibilities. I think that is the first part. (Laughter) Then comes the part where you introduce values and we ask them what are some things that they find important? So they list a whole bunch of things. Then you can choose both objective values vs. subjective values. So objective values are values that anybody in their rational mind (Laughter) would agree is valuable. And subjective values are those, which you know is personal to the client. Not everyone might agree or value the same thing. Yeah, so that's values. And then sometimes when you have a problem is when you have conflict in values. So what you do in situations when you have two objective values in conflict and that is possible, or an objective and a subjective value and you figure out which is more important and then a subjective verses a subjective value. (Laughter)

(T): What are those books, I don't know if you ever used them in school and they were black and yellow? So if you didn't read the book you could go to them.

(P): Cliff notes. (Laughter)

(T): So that was the Cliff notes (Laughter). I will give you the little more lengthy one to fill in some things. You have got the steps and most of the concepts in your mind and that is critically important because really when you do this, if you have the steps and the essential concepts in your mind, then you sort of want to have a discussion or a dialogue with the clients about these ideas. So you can fill in the way you want to fill in, you can back up a little bit; you can do whatever you need to do. I will try to do it with a little more fill in.

You want couples to understand the reasoning. By understanding the meaning of the concepts our mind naturally uses and the relationship of these ideas to one another, it constructs a non-contradictory system of reasoning. The CT is a system of reasoning. By couples discovering through "Socratic dialogue" with a practitioner, these naturally occurring essential concepts, brought to conscious awareness, defining their meaning and then their interrelationships provides humans with the ability to ultimately construct meaning in their life experiences of reality. Further it allows for a universal conceptual form of communication and understanding that has the developmental potential for humans or in this instance couples to be able to resolve conflict in an equitable or just manner.

We do want to begin with reality. And we do want them to be able to understand that we want to have operational definitions for these terms. Because if the mind doesn't understand the concepts it's using, then it can't think as clearly, obviously, and we can't communicate very well if words did not have meaning. That is what Aristotle said. So we know that that is what we want to do, and we might even want to explain to them that this is what it is all about, to be able to communicate and to think more clearly and that means we need to understand the concepts our mind is naturally using. And there are about a dozen concepts our mind, every mind uses, even if it, is unaware of it. Those are the essential concepts of the Conceptual Template. The one term that is used, we are always trying to identify *reality*. Realty is really not a concept. It just is. If we say to them "How do you define that term?" you want them to understand and to say that it just is whatever it is, which is what Aristotle said; what is, is. Then there can be no argument. We don't want to argue with people. Do you know why there can be no argument?

(P): Because it is what it is.(T): Yes, *how can you deny that; reality is whatever it is? What people get into an argument about is how they "see" the reality.*

(P): Or deny reality.

(T): Or deny reality. Good. So often people come in here, and you ask them that question, I often write it down, and (say) don't tell me all about reality. They will tell you all about their metaphysical view of life. You are not interested in that (for this purpose at hand) you are interested in (their understanding) that reality is just is whatever it is. If we can agree on that, then the next step is now we can figure out what it is. So defining reality as that which exists, or that which is, or the nature of things. Those are all fine. Then, at some point we want to get it to their interpretation or *actuality* or how they construct what they are interpreting in reality. But even before that, now I'm doing what you have outlined. You might want to ask them, not might, I think it is critically important, *"Why do we even need to understand reality?"* We want them to understand that it is really important. We do not realize it every day because life is pretty much not difficult in certain ways; it is very difficult in other ways, but we don't have to go out and hunt necessarily, we don't have to go out and fish, we don't have to make a canoe necessarily or a boat. A lot of those things have been done by other great, by other human beings. But they had to figure that reality out too, in order to survive. And *if we do not understand reality sufficiently we cannot survive.*

So often when I am doing this with a couple, I would say something like, you can give any example you want, but I would say, "Let's say you came in my office and I had one of the nurses ...inject a micro-chip in your neck, and I can click it on or off using a transmitter. And I would be able to turn your brain off. What would happen if you left the office and I clicked and turned your brain off? What would happen to you? They might then figure it out. They might fall down the stairs. Some people say they would be wondering around. But ultimately you want to get them to understand, they are not going to live. A lot of couples think you would go to a mental institution, which would be true, but ultimately you are not going to live; you are going to die, because you cannot figure out reality. So you want people to understand that is how serious this can be. And if you are in an emergency situation in life, then you really have to be able to think like that. If you live long enough you may have had a few of those and you realize if I hadn't figured that out I wouldn't be here.

So that is what we want to do. Then we want to start talking about the need to be able to understand reality.

You are doing what when you are thinking about reality? You want to get them to the idea of interpretation. That is the next step. We have a concept for that; we use the word *Actu*ality.

I am probably going to change that to the word *construct* of *reality*. A construct is how the mind puts together whatever it is interpreting or conceptualizing; the mind uses concepts, such as truth. Truth is a concept with regard to reality because we are constructing reality conceptually. Reality just exists, whatever it is. It is not a concept just is what it is. So that is the difference. And once we are interpreting, we need to figure out whether something is *true* or *false* like you said; both are concepts used by the mind to understand or construct reality. And we may have to get the couple to figure that out, the way I have done it with you ... once we experience something, we always *experience reality,* we want to get that point across also. That is what we *experience,* that is what comes through our senses. You can say that sort of thing. But then we need to figure out whether it is <u>blank</u> or <u>blank</u>. It is simple, but people can get confused (but the idea is), to get them to realize it is their interpretation or what is called *Actuality* in the CT, their interpretation or their actuality is either *true* or *false.* Now, we need to define what we mean by something being *true.* The first time you did it you said: "it correlates with reality."

(P): And that wasn't the right word. (Laughter)

(T): That's ok. A lot of people think that because they think correlation is evidence that something is true. It has to have an exact correspondence. And then Yogananda used the word "exact" correspondence. I think that is a good added term.

So something that corresponds exactly to reality well then you know that is the way it is. It is the same with saying the truth. You say that something is and it is, that is the truth. If you say something is, and it is not, that is a false statement. That is how you can hear when people are lying. Well, you just said this. Like you might hear a politician say one thing and then fifteen minutes later totally contradict it, and not realizing they are not telling the truth. And you can tell them over and over, and they do not get it, or they do get it but they don't say they get it. So once we understand that something corresponds, do we really know that it corresponds? So that is when, like you said, that you need to be able to prove, like in science, that what you think is true actually corresponds exactly to reality. It is not just in your mind that it corresponds and that you somehow made something up, and that happens too. You can have exact correspondence in your mind (subjectivity) and it is not true because it is just in your mind so you need something more or less objective, which is the whole idea of this, *learning to be objective.*

And that is a good point. I think you asked me last time, or the time before *"When do you interject the idea of objectivity?" It is real early on, right there. You have to have objective evidence if what you are thinking is true, not just that you think it is true.* I don't know if you can think of examples of that but you might let that roll around in your mind a little bit after today, just to shore things up ... because you can think things correspond and they don't. And you can even have evidence in your mind and it is not true. So you need real objectivity in your thinking and that would lead to knowledge.

And what is knowledge? *Truth is a correspondence between thought and reality, or an exact correspondence; knowledge is a proven correspondence between thought and reality.* Otherwise we don't know or we are not sure, you said. So then the next thing, you know the first part (of the CT) is all about understanding reality that we need to understand just in order to survive and also to have good life. So now we want them to get to the idea, like you were sort of doing, *you might ask people about things that they do. And they tell you, and then you ask them "Why they do it" and they say well I like it or it is important and you want to get them to be able to say something like that. Then you can say, "In other words it is important to you" (has value); people do not always realize that.*

(P): Yeah, from the proof part or the first part to the value (part), like transitioning that. I think I may be missing a little bit of that, a lot (Laughter).

(T): Ok. Again we are trying to bring these essential concepts to a conscious awareness or for the couple to be mindful of these concepts. Buddha used the word mindful; today it is a popularized word. At this point, after the first half of the CT, we want the couple to understand that *values can be defined as that which is important to us and are guiding their (our action).* And sometimes you see people, a couple, one being angry at the other because from their perspective they are doing all the work, their partner is not doing anything, they are just sitting around and are not contributing. When you discuss this with them you find out the reason they don't do something is because they do not like to do whatever it is. They don't value doing it. One person cleans the house and the other person doesn't like doing it. One person does the dishes and the other one doesn't help. One works very hard to make a good living and the other does something that really doesn't help a lot. So, values guide our action. Then once we get that established, we ask them to each make a list of what they value, an extensive list. Couples often come in with only four or five values. You want enough of them (values) in order to differentiate the type of values that they are presenting to you. Then we want them to separate their values into *those things they value on their list (s) that all rational people value, even if they are not aware of it.* That is an important point. For example, people value their health, whether they are aware of it or not. When people are not aware of it, they may do things that are not very healthy. They may make choices that are not very healthy; we all do that at times, obviously. And then we want to separate *values that they value (on their list(s) personally and other rational people may also value, but not necessarily all rational people would value.* So like here in Hawaii, a lot of people value warm weather. To some extent that is a subjective value.

(P): Yeah right, some people like changes in the season, being able to experience snow.

(T): Right, exactly. And where it is very cold human beings have figured out, even in the most difficult of circumstances of cold weather, how to stay warm like the Eskimos, the Inuit. They *know* how to stay warm. They *know* how to survive in that element. Once we have them differentiate these two categories of values, we ask them "What did we just really do?" We separated these values into two categories. You did that right?

(P): Yes.

(T): They are what?

(P): Objective and subjective (values).

(T): Yeah, exactly. And then we said that subjective values could come into conflict with subjective values, objective values in conflict with subjective values, and objective values can be in conflict with other objective values, which is resolved at Stage 6; partly resolved at Stage 5 by the way. You just figure out what is more important in all of those. Objective versus subjective is real simple; which one is more important?

(P): Objective values.

(T): So objective values are always more important than subjective values. And, if you have two subjective values come into conflict it is arbitrary.

(P): Right.

(T): A lot of arguments or fights are about subjective values.

(P): Yeah, because it is how they feel at the time. It can change...

(T): That is a good point. Part of what goes on with human beings is that we often react impulsively to what we want at the moment, or to what we think at the moment. We can also take our time to think about it, examine it, what are the possibilities, and what really makes the most sense in reality, which would be more objective. *It is objectively derived values, because it is derived from reality. Subjectively derived values are derived from our own actuality.*

If we have two subjective values, like you said, it is arbitrary. Objectively derived values coming into conflict is more problematic because they are both objectively of value in reality. So how do you figure that out? One way is to figure out which is more important, again. But sometimes they are equal. They are just equal. So now you have a problem because they are both objective but subjectively different for different people. An example might be the issues of somebody suffering from a horrible disease and in pain all of the time and they no longer want to live. So one person thinks life is objectively of value as the most important thing and therefore they should choose life over euthanasia. Another person who is dying like that may think life is not objectively of value to me now, even though life is of objective value, it is not to me at this time under these life circumstances because I am suffering. So how do you resolve the issue of euthanasia objectively? That is resolved at Stage 6, and partially or even at Stage 5. Any questions?

(P): I remember last week in our last session we talked about these stages and when do you introduce that to the couple.

(T): Yes, you did do that. And that is critically important. And that is done early on. I usually talk to them during the first sessions and again a part of the second session as a review or more specifically about what they heard or understood in the first session, what we are going to do. Or discuss again, to make sure that they understand that we go through cognitive stages of development, how we reason, and cognitive-moral stages or how we reason about what is fair or just. That is sort of how I say it. I might give them an example of cognitive stages, for example we might reason in black or white terms, concretely, and then later in our cognitive development we can think in terms of possibilities or the next stage is thinking in possibilities, more abstractly. People's minds may never develop to that point. Therefore the way they see it, "is the way it is". And then they develop and begin to think in possibilities, well I see it this way but it could be this or that way. That is really a pretty important development in cognition for a human being. Children can't do that. They may be doing it at some level, but not really. It is pretty black or white. Do you know what object permanence is?

(P): Yeah, if they do not see something it is not there.

(T): Yeah that is that kind of idea. They can't think, well, I don't see it and that is why I don't know it is there. They can't do that. You can play that game over and over and be laughing with them for a long time. They don't get it even though every time you do it. You show another possibility.

Then you take them through the moral stages. I sometimes even give them a copy of Kohlberg's stages of moral development. One other thing that is also critically important again is, this is just sort of a discussion with the couple (conversational). You do not have to be perfect. I have been doing this forever, and I am far from perfect. Just like now, I am teaching you this. I am having to comeback or you might have to remind me of something. That might just be me. There might be other people that are doing everything step by step after they read and study the Instructional Manual. When I put the manual together it was from many recordings. The way I was doing it was very linear and not missing too much of anything. If I missed something I would go back. So you give them the stages, explaining them, and then another thing you may want to do is, ought to do, if you want to know if they have developed, you ask them the Slavery Dilemma both at the beginning of counseling (T-1), then you ask them the Slavery Dilemma again (T-2) <u>always</u> *before discussing the concept of value.* You do not want a confounding variable of having discussed objectively and subjectively derived values. Then you can ask them the Slavery Dilemma again, later (T3) etc. after they understand the meaning of objectively derived or based values as distinguished from subjectively based values. This is helpful in determining whether moral development has occurred. Once you have asked them the Slavery Dilemma, you can then ask them other Kohlberg's moral dilemmas such as the Heinz dilemma, although it is not necessary for our purpose, but this is what you would do if you have an interest in identifying their overall moral stage development. Do you know Kohlberg's other moral dilemmas?

(P): No

(T): You can find Kohlberg's moral dilemmas in the appendix of his book *The Psychology of Moral Development*, Volume II.

Ok, you can use the slavery dilemma or substitute slavery with euthanasia. Individuals should write their response on separate sheets of paper so they do not influence each other's answer, actually their *reasoning* for the response. That will tell you right away where they are in their moral development, more or less, specifically if they are Post-conventional. You will know if they are subjective or they are moving toward objectivity, which would be potentially leading to Stage 5 moral reasoning. So you say to them, or give them the following dilemma:

Let's say that in one culture slavery is permitted by their laws, culture, traditions beliefs etc. and therefore they have slavery. In another culture, their laws, traditions, and beliefs prohibit slavery and therefore they do not have slavery.

Is one culture right and the other one wrong, or are they equally right?

Why?

Now they can say whatever they want to say as their answer, which can be content, but *you want to know their moral reasoning or the underlying reasoning for their response. It is the reasoning that is indicative of stage development.* You want to minimally determine if their reasoning is objective or subjective. If it is subjective (personal) they are Conventional Stage 3 or 4 or a mixture even though Conventional moral reasoning can entail objectivity. Pre-conventional is subjectively based and should be, after studying this book be more or less apparent. If they are objective in their moral reasoning they are Post-conventional Stage 5 or 6 or a mixture. If they reject morality, they are relativistic or Pre-conventional. The goal is to facilitate moral development to Post-conventional moral reasoning because it is the most adequate or objective stages of moral reasoning.

Most couples or people are subjective and Conventional in moral reasoning and therefore respond by saying for example, "Both cultures are equally right." When you then ask them "Why?" or for their reasoning, that no one can say what another person or culture ought to do, or what is right or wrong, or it is up to the person or the culture, they might also say something subjective and be at the Conventional level such as, "Well *I personally* believe it is wrong because I am an American or from the United States, or because of or my religion personal beliefs, but no one can say what is right or wrong for another culture or others with different beliefs." They might even say "Everyone has a 'right' to their own beliefs," somehow not realizing the rights of the individuals that are enslaved. There are other possible subjective responses at Stages 3 and 4 such as: "One is right and the other is wrong. It is against my religion." "Or our laws are right and theirs are wrong; slavery is just wrong." "Or, it is just wrong because it hurts people." All of these types of responses have one element in common, which is that the reasoning is subjective. So you would know they are not Post-conventional in their moral reasoning. When a person or couple's moral reasoning is objective, they will give reasons indicative of objectivity by saying one is right and the other wrong giving reasons such as it denies freedom or freedom of choice, or the dignity of the individual or slaves; they would say it is immoral to have slavery under any condition for these objective reasons. In substituting the Euthanasia dilemma, the same holds true. In order to be Post-conventional the reasoning would take into account the individual having rights such as the right to choose what they want to do in these circumstances because life is recognized as being the highest value, or that without life or our existence there would not be values. Individuals have a right to their own decision in this instance because it is their life.

The moral relativist will reject any idea that reflects that there is any objectivity to morality, or will say there is no such thing as moral or immoral. They base their reasoning on the awareness that "no one" agrees on what is moral or what is not, or it is totally subjective and therefore form the more extreme and erroneous conclusion that there is no objective way to say what is moral or immoral; morality has no meaning. This can lead even to the more extreme conclusion that because morality has no meaning, people can do whatever they want.

(P): So what I think for me, what I am not as, I feel like I'm not as good about is, the stages of development. And that is important, trying to move them from one stage to the next, or even gauging what stage they are. And I know that to move them from one stage to the next to use the template, but I am really not very familiar with the stages.

(T): Well I can tell you the stages.

(P): Yeah, I know, I think Stage 2 is good kid bad kid, or about punishment, is that the one?

(T): Stage 1 involves avoiding punishment, getting what one wants, egocentric.

(P): Stage 2 is trying to be the nice person.

(T): That is more characteristic of Stage 3 moral reasoning.

(P): (Laughter) Ok, so I don't have it at all!

(T): No, do you have the chart?

I will explain the stages to you in a simple way.

Stages 1 and 2 are Pre-conventional. I usually make the mistake and say Pre-moral, but it is Pre-conventional and usually it is normally a childhood stage. If adults are in those stages they can be criminals. Incarcerated people, those in jails are commonly Stages 1 and 2. But normally, a child just wants what they want. They try to get what they want. They try to avoid punishment, getting caught or into trouble. You have three children. How old is your youngest?

(P): She is eight. She really tries to avoid getting into trouble.

(T): Stage 2. Now as the mind develops each new stage becomes more adequate than the preceding stage. At the second stage the child or person figures out that one way to get what they want is through some form of reciprocity or exchange; you do this for me and I will do this for you. The third stage might begin when they realize that one way I can get what I want (Stage 2) is by being nice to people.

(P): That is my second daughter.

(T): How old is she, eleven?

(P): Yeah.

(T): That is usually when that kicks in; they are so nice. So Stage 3 is being nice, being a good person. A good boy nice girl orientation that is what it is called. So they are just nice to everybody. It is a great stage. Each stage being more adequate after a while if you are being nice to everybody what happens to you?

(P): They take advantage of you.

(T): Yeah, so then one way to stop that, to being taken advantage of, is to do what?

(P): Oh yeah, that is my son's stage right now. (Laughter)

(T): Yeah, he's like twelve or thirteen?

(P): No, he is fifteen.

(T): So he is learning.

(P): To talk back, standing up for himself, in his mind.

(T): So it could be to avoid or to stop what he considers being taken advantage of …

(P): Right!

(T): He is setting guidelines, rules Stage 4.

(P): Yeah.

(T): Between Stages 2 and 3 it's I can't get what I want, it doesn't work all of the time. I go to school, I want this and they want that. They want my candy bar and say they will give me their sandwich, so they may learn to exchange to get what they want. But after a while that just doesn't work so well, and they figure out to be nice, and now they get it using Stage 3. Some people never get there. You live in a certain environment and it is never being nice that gets you anywhere. Or if it is, it is just enough to manipulate somebody to get what you want. It is not really being nice. So now at Stage 4 it is a rule orientation, and then you might realize at times that rules don't always work. There are certain shows on TV that do that all the time. I think *Law and Order* does this; this is the law but it is not fair and you see them using Stage 5 ... So Stage 5 figures out it doesn't always work if I follow the rule, what is the reason behind the rule? And they start using that; that is Stage 5, the principle or reasoning behind or underlying the rule. And then Stage 6 is even more complicated. Now you have to figure out everybody may have the same rights involved; rights are the principles that underlie Stage 4. If you have a right to something, that would supersede a law. A law is supposed to protect your rights. But sometimes you can have conflicting rights and they are both objectively of value. What do you do? And that is the last part, and I will just say it now. You sort of play "moral musical chairs." You do not know what position you could be in. You could be anybody. And the most important one is the least advantaged position. So what would anybody, not knowing what position they could be in, including the least advantaged position, what would they consider to be fair? So everybody has to figure out well even if I disagree, subjectively, I'd rather be in another position, but objectively I would only want to be in this position that would be objectively fair for anybody, nobody would want to be in the disadvantaged position; it would not be fair. One last point, the stages I described is really simplified but it can give you a sense of each stage. I will give you Kohlberg's description of moral stages.

(P): That was helpful to relate it to my kids, easier to remember.

SESSION 4: CONCEPT OF RIGHTS DEFINED: THE CONCEPT OF RIGHTS IN RELATIONSHIP VALUES AND MORALITY

(T): Last time we talked about a couple of things that might be worthwhile to go over. You asked where to introduce stages, and also the idea of asking that moral dilemma early on as well. So that was productive.

But where we are at, with what is more or less important is through the identification of objectively or subjectively derived values. There is another element here when you think about values or objectively derived values, again what is an objective value beyond just being an objective value?

(P): What do you mean?

(T): Name a couple objective values.

(P): Money.

(T): Ok, what else?

(P): Having shelter.

(T): Ok.

(P): Family.

(T): Ok.

(P): Having relationships with people, health.

(T): So those kinds of values are really what for people? They are their what? I never really know how to introduce this.

(P): Laughter.

(T): I don't. This is when you just have to figure it out, how to get them to understand what you are getting at, and then say it, or sometimes just tell them. Your life, your health.

(P): Necessities.

(T): Necessities, things that you need. They are also your what? It is another word for those things.

(P): Um.

(T): You would not want to be *denied* any of those things. So they are really your what?

(P): Your *rights?*

(T): Very good! I just figured out how to do it. *What you do not want to be denied are your rights.* So that is another way of how you can get into rights; you ask, *"What would you not want to be denied?"* I do use the word denied, or what would you not want to be denied when couples are having trouble figuring out what they value. So it is their rights. You might just have to say, values lead to rights.

(P): Ok.

(T): And then you ask them, like everything else we have done here, we need to figure out what we mean by them (rights) because if we do not understand what something is, how can you really work with it? So what is a right?

(P): Something that you are entitled to? When you are born that everyone should have it.

(T): That is very good. Good for you! That's great. Thomas Paine said something like that, very similar to that. He didn't say like when you were born; I never heard anybody say that. That is really very good. It is something you are *entitled to by virtue of the fact that you exist.*

That is what Thomas Paine said "rights appertain to man in right of his existence" So that tells us a lot.

So now you have rights. Rights entail what? When we have rights that entails what other concepts?

(P): They're all equal.

(T): We might say all rights are equal but they might not always be equal. So when they are not equal then you have what kind of dilemma?

(P): A moral dilemma.

(T): Very good. See, all that I have done here is how can I say something to get you to say what I want you to understand and then to say something, actually anything, that suggests you understand in some way or are making a connection in your own mind of a concept, its meaning, and even its relationship to other concepts that we use to understand whatever we experience or to make sense of what we experience, or to create or construct meaning. Now the Instructional Manual you might want to see what that is. That's very linear, step by step every possibility over many years. Anyway, that is how you do it. You try different things when talking with the couple until they figure it out themselves. A person who is really good at anything can think of a lot of possibilities. And a good psychologist, it is the same thing. You have got to think and figure out if this doesn't work what could work? What is this person thinking (their actuality)? How do I get into their mind?

So this now brings us to the idea (Concept) of *morality*.

(P): Ok.

(T): So now we need to define that.

(P): Right.

(T): So how do rights relate to values? You need to do that also. You just told me rights relate to values in what way?

(P): To objective values, or just values in general?

(T): I asked you just in general, but you can answer that however you want to answer that.

(P): Ok, so rights relate to value, you are entitled to it, you are born with it, and it is important to everyone.

(T): And therefore they must be what kind of values?

(P): *Objective values.*

(T): Right. And so that would even involve subjective values to the extent that everyone has a right to certain subjective values, as long as it does not infringe upon a _____?

(P): Another higher right.

(T): Higher right which would be an objective value or right. But let's say everybody, not everybody; many people have religious beliefs, different belief systems. The reason everybody has a right to religion is because they are subjective; everyone has a right to believe whatever they want to believe. You just cannot impose those beliefs on other people. Now you have got it. So rights are based upon our objective values. And that has to do with when they come into conflict. Whenever you have a conflict between people's interests or claims or rights that is a moral conflict. Now we need to understand what a moral conflict is. What do we mean by the term morality? What does moral mean?

(P): Doing what is right; the difference between right and wrong.

(T): But we realize there are different subjective views.

(P): Yeah, right.

(T): So we're going to define the term. That might be good for you to think about. You had something in your mind. What is morality? I do want to tell you that I have spent many, many, many, many, many moons trying to figure that out. And I figured out what I think is a good answer.

(P): That is a hard question.

SESSION 5: MORAL REASONING AND JUSTICE

(T): Yesterday we talked about the previous session, trying to get a sense of what this is all about, which is important for a person whose doing this, to grasp. It is critical that people realize that identifying reality is important in their life. I think a lot of people don't. And, then once understanding that, part of that reality is making decisions, and those decisions generally are sometimes not made in a conscious way with regard to it being more objective or subjective. I thought about that a little bit. Then it was talked about how we could have an objective and a subjective decision come into conflict, or two objective values come into conflict, or we could have two subjective decisions conflicting. Sometimes you might have an objective and subjective value and you think now I have got to do the objective one; that might be a pretty boring life sometimes. So I think it is up to the individual but in my particular way of thinking, in my life, there are times there is something clearly objective, what I should be doing, and subjective that probably would not be such a "good decision" from some standpoint.

Like, for example, something might be little dangerous objectively. And so you might think, maybe I shouldn't do that because objectively it is dangerous, but maybe it is a lot of fun to do that part of it being dangerous. Objectively jumping out of a plane, skydiving is probably not quite as safe as walking on the ground but if you like the idea of flying through the air you might, well, I am willing to take that chance for, you could say, my objective happiness. The idea of you doing this is to have a grasp of all of it, figuring it out in your own mind in some way you are aware of it, so you can present this in a way that you can be somewhat spontaneous when you are working with a couple and even make mistakes and come back to it, and figure it out. A couple other things we talked about that are critically important that you asked before, "When do you introduce the idea of objectivity?" I would say right around when we are *interpreting, the concept of Actuality, the second Step,* being objective about, "Is what I am thinking true or false?" so early on in the CT. The other thing I recommended to you was to ask the moral dilemma about slavery. If you don't want to use the slavery dilemma for some reason, than you can switch it to euthanasia or you could use both. You just want to find out if they are subjective in their moral reasoning/judgment. If they are subjective in their reasoning of the slavery dilemma, then they are not at Stage 5, or Post-conventional. They can't be, so their reasoning tells you right away. And that way, I don't think I mentioned this to you either, that later on, when you are done or think you are done with the couple, or you think or don't think they are more developed, you can ask the dilemma questions to them again. So now you have an objective measurement that they have or have not actually developed. And then we went on to what kind of values there are. We differentiated objectively derived values, based upon reality, and subjectively derived values that are based on our own actuality. Lastly we talked a little bit more about ...

(P): Rights.

(T): Rights. I sort of led you into that. I have never been able to get people into that easily. I said to you *"What would you not want to be denied?"* I never thought of that before. I have used that idea when I wanted people to get more values written down than they had. It was easier for them than "What do you value?" But that can lead to rights too; that was what you said was difficult for you, to make that transition. People realize that they do not want to be denied what they want, value, or maybe that to which they have a right. I don't know. I don't have an answer for that one. But, you want to get them into rights. You defined rights as ...

(P): What you are entitled to.

(T): Because of born or something like that.

(P): Born, yeah.

(T): Yeah, which I told you I have never heard anybody say that. But, Thomas Paine said that rights are that which you are entitled to by virtue of your existence. So that is the same idea. And that is very good. The fact that we exist puts us all on a real even universal basis.

(P): Uh hum.

(T): What would any of us think, that because we exist, we ought to have (as a right). For example, like education. Some people might think we do not have a right to it or to a good education, but anybody who is born needs to be educated. It is a need, not even a want. Needs, both physical and metaphysical needs such as freedom are our rights. Needs and wants can be differentiated that way also, just to mention it. Subjective values are more like wants or desires and objectively derived values are based upon needs. We all need to be educated. Some people may not realize that. You could say if having lived in a culture like here (Hawaii) many years ago or even on some of the smaller islands, you might need to know how to make a boat. It is an education. Or like learning to climb up a tree, that's an education. So we all *need* an *education*. Looking at rights from the standpoint of we exist, what do we need, then we have those values that are all objectively based in reality. So we got to rights. Then we sort of sped up a little bit. I thought we were going a little fast. So let's just go into the next concept. I asked you what area, I don't know how to say this to people either, but what domain are rights in? You did say it yesterday. You know that right? If we are talking about, if I said to you what domain is this in food, shelter, water you would say it is in what domain? They are our, <u>blank</u>?

(P): Our needs.

(T): Yeah. If I said ice-skating, going to movies, weightlifting, that would be in what sort of domain?

(P): Our likes.

(T): Our likes, right, which are subjective, but they are our likes. If we talk about the idea of rights, what domain is that in? When we talk about rights, what is that all about? You said it yesterday.

(P): I did?

(T): Yeah, you did.

(P): When we talk about our rights, what domain? What does it mean?

(T): We are talking about, you are telling me you have a right, I am saying I am denying you that right, that is what kind of issue?

(P): What kind of issue?

(T): Yeah, if I deny you your rights and you say you have a right to that, not like a child saying it, but as an adult. Let say a human being feels they have a right and they are being denied that right that is what kind of an issue, what domain is that in?

(P): Our entitlements.

(T): So we are entitled to something and somebody denies it, it becomes what kind of an issue, what kind of conflict is that?

(P): Our personal, I don't know.

(T): If someone denies you your right they are basically being what to you?

(P): They deny me my right?

(T): Yeah that you have a right to something. Let's say you are married.

(P): My freedom.

(T): Your freedom, right! So that is your right, your freedom, and your rights. If somebody says you can't be free, they are really being what to you? If I deny you your freedom, if the government denies you your freedom, there are governments that do, they are being.

(P): Controlling.

(T): Yeah, they are being controlling but they are also being what to you? It is what? You would say it is what? You might say to your husband that you are doing the dishes every night, you are doing the cleaning, you are doing all these things, you also work, and he doesn't do it. You would say he is being what?

(P): An (expletive) (Laughter)

(T): Yeah that's true. (Laughter) That will be redacted. Yeah, he is being "An (expletive)" to you because he is being what to you?

(P): Like a tyrant.

(T): He is being like a tyrant. He is being what? He is treating you in what way?

(P): He is being mean.

(T): Being mean to somebody might be what?

(P): Disrespectful.

(T): Disrespectful, but if he doesn't allow you to do certain things like he does, and it is not equal, than it is.

(P): Authoritarian.

(T): Yeah he's being authoritarian. Just so you know, in psychology, basically there is no such thing as authoritarianism. I totally disagree. There is a psychologist, Rokeach who wrote a book called the *Authoritarian Personality*. Ok, if someone is not treating you equally, he or she is not being what?

(P): Unfair.

(T): Unfair. All right, *so you might have to go through all this with people to get what you want them to understand.* And you can tell (identify) that people can get real frustrated when they might for example, "What do you want me to say?" (Laughter)

(P): Yeah.

(T): But you have got to get them to say it.

(P): Unfair?

(T): Yeah.

(P): Ok.

(T): So when we talk about fairness or unfairness, we are in what domain? What is that called? What category is that in? Do you know the concept for that?

(P): No.

(T): Morality.

(P): Oh. I don't know how it is related.

(T): How morality.

(P): Is related to being fair or unfair.

(T): *What is morality all about? That was your assignment.* Ok. So we are in the domain of morality about fairness. The question I asked you yesterday was how would you define moral or morality? What is that all about? We didn't have time to think about that with all that goes on in your life. That is why the great thinkers were called armchair philosophers. At that time they came from wealthy families. They could sit around and think about things, figure things out. Most of us don't seem to have time for that, unless you go to school for that.

(P): So we're talking about how it's related to being fair.

(T): No, no I just started to ask you, you said it wasn't.

(P): Well I said I didn't know how you were trying to relate the two.

(T): Right, it's hard to figure this out.

(P): Yeah.

(T): Even if you have to give people some of this stuff, I don't think it is a bad thing. In some way that is the finesse you have to have to figure it out or help couples to discover the concepts their mind naturally uses to actually understand their experiences in order to survive and to thrive. Most people don't even know if you give it to them. They can also question and even reject what you say, in some sense that should be encouraged. A couple does not usually do that because couples sometimes come to a practitioner, psychologist, a social worker, or what have you because we're supposed to know ... be an authority. The purpose of the CT and the use of a "Socratic" method or process facilitate rationality, objectivity, a respect for truth, relevant evidence, understanding or knowledge and as such it encourages autonomy of thought through an inherent respect for reason rather than a belief even in the "authority" of a practitioner. Reason is the "authority." Sometimes I will ask the couple. "Who is the authority in here?" and if they say that I am the authority, I will ask them again and again until they figure out that it is their innate ability to reason, and that being mindful of learning to be objective in their reasoning is the "authority."

Ok, so back to yesterday, I did ask you when we were talking about morality, "What is morality all about?"

(P): Well I feel like morals are like guidelines for behavior. For good and bad, right and wrong.

(T): Ok. Right. Ayn Rand, do you know who she is? You might want to read something of hers. Like the novel *Atlas Shrugged*; it is really a great book. I don't know if she considered that her masterpiece; she also wrote other books. A lot of the smartest people I have known as women and thinkers ahead of their time have read Ayn Rand. They are just very rational. But I have seen them be pretty irrational too. I have seen Ayn Rand being pretty irrational; we are all irrational at times. So Ayn Rand defined morality similar to the way you did. You said guidelines to our behavior. She said morality is a code of values that guide our choices and actions ... I would have to look it up, but that is close to what you are saying right?

(P): Objective values, objectively derived values.

(T): Well it should be objectively derived values that guide our choices and actions and that is morality. If we treat someone unfairly, is that a moral issue?

(P): Yeah, it is because, well it depends upon the consequences.

(T): If you are treating somebody unfairly...

(P): But maybe you have to, maybe they feel like it is unfair, but it is fair so that means equal right?

(T): What does fairness mean? That is going to be another issue. See, that is a natural question. So if you said that later I would say fairness has to do with whether or not something is equal, being equitable. So, the great thinkers at least Western, I am sure Eastern as well, saw the issue of justice as the main issue of morality, having to do with justice. If something is just or it is unjust in the way we treat other people, and that was under the domain of morality. So what you said about morality is good enough, how we treat other people, is it right or wrong, you didn't use the word fair or unfair, but maybe that isn't a word you would use for that, but it would be a word that could come up later on; it just came up.

(P): Right. (Laughter)

(T): Right. I thought you said

(P): Yeah.

(T): Yeah, so morality has to do with we, what did you say, again?

(P): The way we behave.

(T): Yeah the way we behave, whether it is right or wrong.

(P): Yeah.

(T): And then you just said that has to do with objective values.

(P): Yeah.

(T): Which is good. Because if you look at the way morality is in reality, it may not be as objective as people think it is. Like we talked yesterday, for a moment about the Spanish Inquisition .... They thought that was moral, that that was good. And we see that today... You brought up ISIS. They viewed what was moral in one way and other people viewed it in another.

(P): How they treat women.

(T): Yeah. So things contradict. Something cannot both be and not be at the same time. Something cannot both be good and bad at the same time. So something is "rotten in Denmark." There has to be some consistent logic or orientation in thinking or reasoning, *moral reasoning that* we can all agree is fair or just to everybody. The only way to do that is to determine those things that are <u>Blank</u>.

(P): How do we determine something is fair/just to everyone?

(T): Yeah, we would have to be what about it?

(P): Objective.

(T): Yeah, we would have to be objective. It would have to be the same for you, me and everyone else. So in the Me Too Movement today, women are saying you are not treating us equally, you are not paying us the same for doing the same job. Some of us have a better education then our male counterparts, that is unfair, that is immoral. They all sort of go together. At least according to, I can't think of anybody who thinks like that unless they are being subjective. So morality has to do with our behavior in terms of our underlying *moral reasoning*, how we treat other people and whether or not it is "right or wrong." And the only way we can have something consistent that everybody can agree upon is to find those things that are objectively of value to all people. So there are some things like that. For example, you could say the Ten Commandments are objective; thou shalt not kill, thou shall not steal, thou shall not bare false witness against thy neighbor, etc. They seem pretty good, except there is a problem (besides the listed Commandment being incorrectly stated or not in the correct order). So that is where we want to learn something else. And so you would say something like that, to couples if they were operating at Stage 4 or any kind of rule orientation. For example, during Nazi Germany, in an apartment building, and the Nazi's come, the Gestapo, and they start coming in doing whatever they are going to do, they did a lot of bad things. They go upstairs; they try to find somebody but that person is not there. They go back down to you, you are on the first floor, and they ask you: "Did you see them leave because we want to talk to them?" You did see them leave and you could tell them which way they went so you could tell them the truth or you could lie. If you tell them the truth the consequences are obvious.

(P): Right.

(T): They would be taken to a concentration camp, and probably be killed. People knew that. So what would you do? I'll tell you a quick story after this. Would you tell them the truth?

(P): No you would lie.

(T): Being honest is the same idea, as thou shalt not steal. Right? Sorry for giving you a stealing example, but that is the same idea although honesty is not one of the Ten Commandments.

(P): Well you can relate it to current events, with ICE and the illegal immigrants. They are searching them out now in towns and cities and into people's homes and their workplace. They are looking for illegal immigrants who have been here for years, trying to get rid of them. It is really relevant currently.

(T): So we were talking about morality, being fair or just.

What is that all about? That is the next concept. People like Socrates talked about the idea (concept) of justice. That is the main issue. If you think about it (justice), if we treat people fairly, that is of value, to everybody, then how do you figure that out? Well, it could be figured out that we have *rights*. Having rights is the underlying moral reasoning for our laws. That is at Stage 5.

That is what you hear. People are talking about individual rights superseding somebody else's laws or what have you. For example, somebody stops at a red light and then goes through to save somebody's life. The police want to put them in jail for running a red light. The judge makes a judgment saying they were using their right to life that superseded the law. The moral reasoning of law is to or is supposed to protect a human life. It is not that they just ran it. They stopped, they looked, they made sure that nobody was there, and then they ran the red light. So where the letter of the law does not work, (Stage 4) *principles* or the reasoning behind the laws (Stage 5) are more adequate in determining what is fair or just.

And a principle is, this you just have to sort of teach couples or clients so you are just going to have to try to remember it. A *principle* is not like a principle as meaning a strong conviction. It really basically means that it has to meet two criteria philosophically. One is that it is *reversible*. Which means if I were in your shoes or you were in my shoes we could both accept the resolution as being fair or just; nobody is going to want something that is going to be unfair to them. So if we both can agree if I put myself in your shoes or vice versa, and we can agree that it is fair then we have reversibility. The second one is called universalizability, which is a countercheck of reversibility. And it says, even if one subjectively disagrees, they can't rationally/objectively disagree that the principle works; that it is equitable, equally fair/just to both of us. I don't know that I can give you a good example of that now. But that is what Stage 6 moral reasoning figures out. But you could also say if I have a right to something, then you ought to have a right to something and vice versa. So that would work in terms of reversibility. And even if one of us disagreed with that right, we could not deny under the "veil of ignorance" (Rawls, 1971, pp. 136–142) that the right was fair. Let's say a person thought that women are not equal to men. But if we said well "if you were a woman or a man or you would not know if you were to be a man or a woman, how would you think then?" That idea, again like "moral musical chairs" if you don't know, if you were to be born a woman or a man, how would you think, you would think a man and a women are equal and should be treated equally.

(P): She would agree with that.
(T): Yeah well of course, it is fair. But some could say: "I disagree, women need to know their place." That kind of idea sounds absurd when I say it like this, but for some people it doesn't sound absurd.

(P): I mean you could take the immigration issue right?

(T): Yeah.

(P): I don't believe immigrants should be here even though they have been here for twenty years. But if you were in that position would you want to be deported back to a country where you don't even know anymore. I mean you were raised here. You came here when you were a child.

(T): Yeah a better example. So you are better at doing that then I am. My mind is packed with...

(P): Disorderly. (Laughter)

(T): Yeah. That is the idea of it. That is Stage 5 or 6. Stage 6 can figure out or construct the moral reasoning that if you don't know which position you are (could be) in ... It is called *"moral musical chairs"*, is one way to put it, or a *veil of ignorance*. When we see that statue, the one with the two, or a scale, like a balance and the blindfold over the eyes it represents that veil of ignorance. If you can't tell who you are going to be in a situation, that is what Stage 6 moral reasoning figures out. You could be anybody in that situation, but most importantly it has to include the "least advantaged" individual. And then you figure out or your moral reasoning would understand that I wouldn't, nor would any rational person want to be in that position. Or I wouldn't want to be sent back to where I was born after all this time. You know, our President, who might say that, he couldn't rationally disagree that if you are in that position, he wouldn't want to be sent back either. Especially if he knows that most probably he is going to die because you left that country.

(P): Right.

(T): Or they're still that way. There are parts of the world that you go back and they are very dangerous.

(P): Or you don't have any family there.

(T): Or you don't have anything there.

(P): You don't speak the language, nothing.

(T): Right. So that is how we can figure things out that are fair to everybody and that is Stage 6 moral reasoning. And that is what justice is. Justice treats everyone equally, equitably.

(P): Even if you don't agree?

(T): Even if you don't agree subjectively. There can be two objectively based positions but having a subjectively different preference.

(T): I think you understand it pretty clearly, right?

(P): Uh Hugh.

(T): Ok. I think that is basically it. And what I did with you yesterday was sort of quick. But you understand it.

(P): Uh Hugh.

(T): I can tell. And that is the same thing when you are working with somebody you might have to do something like this. It was easy with you to understand this form of reasoning, namely, what I just said with regard to what is fair and just. But for other people they don't know or understand or grasp that form of moral reasoning or what you are talking about. They cannot put themselves in the shoes of another. I think you can think of some people today that they just can't do that.

(P): Yeah, especially working with couples. They are so stuck in their own subjectivity they cannot see beyond what is fair for the other person; they are so angry and emotional.

(T): Right. So you know again a good example might be good for you to do. You know that is the one thing that I also see with couples. And the thesis of everything I am doing with this book has to do with that. The one thing that creates real serious issues with couples is being treated or perceiving that they are being treated unfairly.

(P): Uh hum.

(T): There are other things that affect a marriage. But when you have people treating each other fairly, it definitely, I know that, because I have done it, maybe knowing it is a strange word to use here, perhaps having the moral reasoning capability is better, but it certainly clearly appears that people who develop to the fifth stage, even if they get divorced, treat the other person more fairly and so they are treating each other the same when they are getting divorced. So it may not be that they will stay together, but you see it all the time that a lot of the fights …

(P): Yeah, and that is good, because I have never taken it that far where to have them reverse roles or think about the other person, you know if they were in that position, how would they feel?

(T): And you used the word "role" here. Role taking. There is a professor, Robert Selman, if you look up "role taking" you would see it, he is at Harvard. His whole thesis is about role taking, his work is significant, he was right. When I was there knowing him I didn't think it was a big deal, I didn't know why everybody made such a big fuss, or Kohlberg in particular, about role taking, but the more I learned, and even after I graduated, I began to realize, he was right on target. If you can't put yourself in the shoes of another, or having empathy … So you might want to look at that some time, Robert Selman, that is his name.

(P): *It is not just putting your shoes in another and still being subjective but it is really putting yourself in another person's shoes and being objective, looking at objective values and rights.* Because it is easy to be like, well if I were in her position I wouldn't feel that way because I would be fine with me working and bringing in the money.

(T): Exactly. And in fact in a journal article I wrote, I did use that kind of example of putting yourself in the shoes of another, how would you feel? Most people say…

(P): They would be fine with it. Yeah it is happening right now under this administration.

(T): Yeah, there are a lot of people that I know that are very highly intelligent successful people and they do not have a problem with any of it. The reason they do not have a problem with it, is because of what they value. They are all very successful people. They make a really good living, men and women, by the way. They know he is a businessman, and he is going to do this, our stocks are going to go up, I am going to look out for me. If you do not look out for yourself, in a certain way, you are a fool. And they tell me that, more or less, the one's who know me closely enough. They will tell me that, "What is wrong with you?" Why didn't you charge 300 dollars an hour? You could have. ... I just didn't do that. I think 150 is a lot, even to this day. It would have been a big difference when I saw forty, fifty or sixty people a week. I would be in a different position then I am now. But I am not sorry that I did what I did. It depends on what you value and your moral reasoning that guides your actions. What are people's rights that you take into account in your moral judgment? Putting yourself in the position of another, role taking, not knowing what position you could be, how would you want it to be even if you subjectively were to disagree? It is real clear. Having a basic understanding of what is fair or just and being able to use the concepts ... it is really pretty wonderful; how could it not be? If somebody treats you fairly ... but, there are people who could be at Stage 5, and they still, because of emotional issues react to something and they cannot do it until later. To draw this to a close, we react to things, ... we do not stop, think, reflect and then chose to act. I think our brains are innately wired that way because at one time we had to just react, but today people still can react ...

(P): And they don't realize it; it is so automatic.

(T): It is so automatic, right.

(P): So if they just learn to just pause and think or reason objectively they would avoid some conflict. (Laughter)

(T): Avoid a lot of conflict! (Laughter)

(P): Especially with couples.

(T): Especially with couples.

Chapter 13

Discussion

Lawrence Kohlberg

As mentioned in the Introduction, the last thing Kohlberg said to me after graduation was "Go out there and do this!" I was living in Chicago when I next heard from him. He was in Chicago, I believe, to visit a close friend of his at the University of Chicago. Our phone conversation was personal, intimate, and reminiscent of a conversation we had in his office when it appeared to be a fait accompli that I would be accepted into the doctoral program in clinical psychology. His demeanor was quietly still. He told me, when sitting alone together, that he did not know if he could stay alive long enough that he would be able to work with me to the completion of my doctorate in moral education. He explained that he had an intestinal infection caused by a giardia parasite and was often experiencing what I interpreted as anguishing pain. The implication was clear, and not really knowing what to say, I paused, and he then said he would do his best if I were willing. I said yes to this verbal contract with the silent thought that our understanding/agreement was just. What has been until now personal and never said before, is mentioned here with the intention that it might give the readers a glimpse into Larry's character. I believe that it can, in this context, give others insight into his dedication to life-long research, and his efforts to continue his life for the sake of others, and in this particular instance, his student(s). He was authentic and sincere. He was a teacher, dissertation committee chairman, a mentor in the truest sense of the meaning of this word, and, to me, a caring and loving friend. He frequently appeared to be experiencing pain and to suffer mentally from medication that just would not cure him, yet we had an unspoken trust for one another, we continued to work together. And again, as indicated in the Introduction, there appeared to be both an explicit and implicit understanding and trust of one another, that I did not, nor did he, find to be unusual with others. I tell you all of this so that it will be understood what I would next like to clearly convey to those who did not know this often quiet, reserved, introspective and sometimes disheveled, genius.

I do not use the word genius loosely. I use the term because it speaks to the truth and significance of what Kohlberg has provided to humanity, to all of us. His life's work in moral development, for those who knew him, even those who intelligently challenged him in some areas of his theory, could not but help to have the utmost respect because of what he had done over his lifetime.

He has provided a paradigm of moral development that just so happens to have answered my life-long questions regarding human social interaction, "Why do people do the things they do?" Or more accurately, "Why, or what are the *reasons*, that *we all* do the things we do?" And, "What are the reasons that some would want to harm another or others?" Of course, these were initially the questions of an innocent child that perseverated in this form of questioning, to some extent, until this day. Lawrence Kohlberg's longitudinal research on moral development answered these interrelated questions. And for this reason, I think it is a responsibility to those who do not realize the monumental implications or significance of Kohlberg's research to inform them. In the Introduction, in the context of mentioning other great thinkers, such a Socrates, Plato, Aristotle, I intentionally and appropriately mentioned, in the same breath of life, Lawrence Kohlberg, because of his contribution to a better understanding of moral development and its profound significance for humanity, for all of us.

Kohlberg has provided us with an understanding of morality and justice, explained in a manner that is evidence based, and practical. He explains that morality cannot, as historically defined by Aristotle, be understood as virtuous behavior. This is because what is considered virtuous, although perhaps at times appears to be admirable, is nonetheless viewed in various ways, and can be inconsistent across differing circumstances, or is limited because of its specificity. Kohlberg depicts morality as a cognitive and cognitive-moral developmental process of reasoning. Moral judgment/reasoning develops in an invariant, universal sequence of stages. Each stage is more adequate in resolving conflict, or conflicting claims or interests, than the preceding stage with respect to justice concerns. The least developed stages are *self-centered*. The most developed stage, Post-conventional Stage 6, is a construct of moral reasoning that is *all encompassing* when objectively understood; it would be agreeable to any rational mind when used to resolve issues of what is considered just to *all* involved, *including the least advantaged person(s)*. And further, even if there is subjective disagreement with others, the use of this construct of moral reasoning can nevertheless be rationally, and in a non-contradictory manner, be objectively proven to be equally just for all involved.

What Kohlberg has provided humanity is a framework of moral development. Stages of moral development or stages of moral judgment/reasoning can be objectively identified or described, as can their universal invariant sequence, from less adequate to most adequate constructs of resolving a conflicting claim or interest in a just manner, thus lending itself to being measurable. The stages are associated with, or related to, how individuals behaviorally treat one another in matters concerning that which is just (Blasi, 1980). Rational, reasonable people can objectively agree that the least developed stages of moral reasoning and associated behaviors are clearly less adequate in resolving conflicts of interest or claims in a just manner than are the more developed stages of moral judgment. In a parallel way, rational, reasonable and objectively reasoning individuals can agree that more developed stages of moral reasoning, and their associated behaviors are clearly more adequate. Kohlberg has actually provided humanity, in reality, with a "moral compass," in its truest sense of its meaning. We now understand, or know, having a proven correspondence between Kohlberg's thought and reality, and based upon empirical research or objective scientific observation/evidence, that moral judgment/reasoning is developmental, or in his own words:

> Our research shows that individual development in moral reasoning is a continual differentiation of moral universalizability from more subjective or culturally specific habits or beliefs While moral behaviors or customs seem to vary from culture to culture, underneath these variations in custom there seem to be universal kinds of judging or valuing. Sexual mores obviously vary widely by culture and historical epoch, even if norms about life and property less clearly vary. This variation in sexual customs does not necessarily imply, however, differences in basic moral values or ways of judging. The culturally variable customs of monogamy and polygamy are both compatible with the culturally universal underlying moral norms of personal dignity, commitment, and trust in sexual relationships.
>
> (Kohlberg, 1984)

When Kohlberg said me to "Go out there and do this!" he was implicitly, if not explicitly, expressing that it is important for counseling therapists, psychologists, educators, and, most importantly, humanity to realize the implications and therefore the significance of his research in moral development. At the same time, he was directly encouraging me to use the "Conceptual Template" (CT) as a pragmatic application of providing a means by which to facilitate moral development to the Post-conventional level. Writing this book is, for one, a step in that direction. But to reify what is important for those having an interest in Kohlberg's stages for its use in couples therapy is to also realize the monumental achievement in what Kohlberg has provided for all of us, and potentially for all of humanity. The application of this new Conceptual Template approach to couple therapy, having its foundation in Kohlberg's research, is one way, with the utmost of respect, to honor Lawrence Kohlberg himself.

He encouraged, or admonished me in his own way to apply the "Conceptual Template" to the question somewhat paradoxically left unanswered in his research. This question was how to facilitate moral development to Post-conventional moral reasoning.

An understanding of Kohlberg's theory has been emphasized throughout this book, as it was his longitudinal empirical research of moral development (Kohlberg, 1958) that served as the theoretical foundation to this approach to couple therapy. This approach, guided by the couple therapist, fosters the discovery of a system of reasoning, the construction of what is now referred to as the Conceptual Template (Ries, 1979, 1981, 1992/2006).

The Conceptual Template is a system of reasoning representing a conceptually integrated and logically consistent approach to thinking rationally, objectively, and clearly. With the guidance of a couple therapist, individuals discover the Conceptual Template for themselves through a Socratic dialogue and then can apply this conscious-awareness or mindfulness to any decisions in their experiences of life, including moral experiences. Use of this system of reasoning was found to facilitate not only moral development in general, but more specifically, Post-conventional moral reasoning (Ries, 1981/1992/2006). It was later observed in clinical practice that facilitating moral development paralleled an improvement in couples or marital relationships.

Kohlberg was attempting to understand an anomaly in moral development during the time that I worked with him. Several of his subjects in his longitudinal study appeared to regress in their moral reasoning. However, this apparent regression was found to actually be a period of reflective questioning often associated with identity confusion, and relativism, but also, critically significant, a potential transition to Post-conventional Stage 5 moral reasoning. Determining how to facilitate this *"potential"* transition to a higher level of moral reasoning, namely, Post-conventional Stage 5 and 6, peaked my interest.

During informal research of this potential transition, Kohlberg's subjects were observed by the author to share a commonality during this period of reflective questioning and potential transition: they were concerned with and confused about specific issues surrounding the inadequacy of their earlier Stages 3 and 4 moral reasoning. The manifestation of this recognition appeared in the form of particular types of questions or concerns. These concerns consistently focused upon questions such as, "Who am I?" "What is the meaning of my existence?" "What is reality?" In asking these types of questions, these individuals appeared to be also consistently focusing upon the ideas of truth, knowledge, objectivity, subjectivity, opinion, belief, values, good and evil, morality and justice. It appeared to me that these individuals focused upon specific questions and ideas in order to untangle their confusion and then reconstruct meaning in their lives.

Preliminary research (Ries, 1979), of autobiographies and some biographies, such as those of Carl Gustav Jung, Anais Nin, Martin Luther King among others, found that when these individuals experienced a similar transitional period, they, like Kohlberg's subjects, were concerned with the same questions regarding the same specific issues of truth, knowledge, objectivity, subjectivity, belief, opinion, values, morality and justice. It occurred to me that philosophers, or great thinkers, seemed to share this commonality of questions and concerns. They too, were concerned about these same issues, and spent much time attempting to resolve, define and interrelate these particular concepts. Thus, using the specific ideas or essential philosophical concepts that were common and recurrent among philosophers, Kohlberg's subjects, as well those in my preliminary research studies, I began to construct a paradigm, using the teachings of Socrates, Plato, and Aristotle into a unified conceptual framework which is systematic and non-contradictory, and that can be used to think more clearly, rationally, logically and objectively about one's own thinking, reasoning or interpretation of reality. It can be applied to more adequately interpreting another's form or reasoning, as well. The hypothesis was that learning, or discovering for one's self, concepts that appear essential to rational thought in an integrated form (which can naturally occur in human development, as a cognitive-developmental or rational thought process) can lead to an understanding of life which is more intelligible and non-contradictory and thereby facilitate moral development as defined by Kohlberg's cognitive-moral developmental theory. The findings of a double blind study (1981, 1992/2006) testing this hypothesis found that the use of this system of reasoning, which contained essential philosophical concepts (presently referred to as the Conceptual Template), significantly facilitated moral development in general, and in particular, Post-conventional (Stage 5) moral reasoning. This Post-developmental moral reasoning aligns with development from the antecedent concept of self in the particular, or a subjective social role identity, to a more objective universal concept of self (Ries, 1981, 1992/2006). As mentioned earlier, it was later observed that using this same approach in counseling indicates a parallel between moral development and the improvement of relationships.

Chapter 14

Conclusion

The purpose of this book is to present a unique approach for couple or marital counseling which can be used alone or in conjunction with other approaches. It is unique in that it does not suggest or tell couples what to do or how to improve their relationships. Rather, the intervention is to teach couples, in a Socratic manner, how to discover for themselves, by becoming consciously aware, mindful or knowledgeable, how their minds can work conceptually, and further, how applying this framework, the Conceptual Template, can guide them toward resolving most issues or concerns they might have, as well as enhance their ability to relate more intimately as a couple. "Give a man a fish, and you have fed him once. Teach him how to fish and you have fed him for a lifetime." Rather than giving a couple fish, they learn to fish.

Couples relationships involves contact, understanding and communication. When having interaction with one another, we can miscommunicate or misunderstand one another because, for one, our actual experiences or interpretation of a reality may differ. Further, we can misunderstand the meaning of words, how they are meant, or how others use them. All of these factors, among others, can lead to conflict. The concepts in the Conceptual Template give definition, concreteness or conscious meaning to specific words or concepts and their interrelationships that the mind naturally uses in order to understand our experiences of reality, of one another, and of the choices we then make. The value of being mindful or having knowledge of this natural process that the brain already innately uses to interpret, construct, or understand any reality in either the non-moral or moral realm of human experience, is that the better we understand and are consciously aware of this natural occurring process, the more adequately we can utilize it. The better the understanding of how our minds "work" or conceptually process experiences, the more adequately we can then understand reality, and respond or make choices that are rational, consistent and non-contradictory to our well-being. Giving definition and meaning to these concepts and their interrelationships makes them concrete and gives us knowledge of the natural processes that the brain innately uses. By being mindful of the conceptual thought process, the Conceptual Template can be a guide or standard by which a couple can consciously treat one another in an equitable and just manner, thereby improving their relationship.

There is no panacea for improving couples or marital relationships. There are many factors that affect couples; however, these other factors can be at least tempered by an awareness of a rational thought process or those concepts necessary for objective reasoning, particularly as this process pertains to our subjective and relativistic constructs of that which is considered just. Conflict that couples have when choosing to have therapeutic assistance invariably involve one or both individuals feeling or thinking that they are being treated unfairly. The cause of injustice is that one or both individuals is morally subjective (subjectivism) or morally relativistic (relativism). The resolution to conflict or injustice is moral objectivism. The Conceptual Template process is an approach to couple therapy, which can result in resolving conflicting claims or interests objectively. Kohlberg's invariant sequence of moral stage development is both a measure and countercheck to a clinical assessment of meaningful change particularly as it relates to couples' behavioral interactions.

The Conceptual Template reveals a universal thinking process through the identification, conceptualization, and integration of specific and essential philosophical concepts or ideas. It provides a logical, systematic and non-contradictory approach to improving the natural ability to think more rationally and objectively. It teaches an objective thinking process that can enhance critical thinking skills. And, the Conceptual Template can facilitate moral development in general, and in particular, post-conventional reasoning and moral judgment (Stages 5 and 6). In essence the Conceptual Template empowers couples or individuals with a consistent, non-contradictory, and rational means of understanding one another and applying their reasoning ability to problem solving and decision making in a manner that is equitable. Ultimately this conceptual mindfulness results in improving communication, trust and intimacy in couples' relationships.

The objectives of this new and useful approach to improving couple relationships are:

a   To teach individuals how to apply the Conceptual Template to enhance their own development and their relationships through objective thinking.
b   To enable couples to create a healthier relationship based upon mutual respect and understanding.
c   To help couples apply essential concepts necessary for both objective as well as rationally consistent reasoning.
d   To appreciate the concept of the *faculty of reason* and *rational thought* as an innate natural process that can be improved as a skill and then applied to crisis situations.

e   To appreciate moral reasoning. How we should treat and be treated by others is extremely important for couples to understand.

f   To enable relationships to grow through reasoning in a rational, logical, consistent, and non-contradictory manner and to express comfort, intimacy and love.

g   To teach couples to apply this process of morally focused thinking and being to all aspects of life that require trust and communication.

h   To support individuals in understanding their natural ability to think, communicate and resolve differences fairly.

i   To enable couples to learn to be consciously aware or mindful of these processes so that they can quickly resolve conflict to their mutual satisfaction.

As couples move toward a higher level of moral development and reasoning, they become more satisfied with one another. By enhancing moral reasoning (cognitive and cognitive-moral development), the couple, as a team, will be more resilient, with the resources necessary to thrive (not just survive) traumatic events and lesser challenges. Just as an individual makes an effort to evolve in moral development, couples struggle to evolve in their trust and understanding with one another. This is essential for true intimacy. Just as distinct stages of moral reasoning follow a pattern that emerges as a moral foundation for life choices, so too are couple relationships built. Common knowledge and experience in relationships suggest that it is important for couples to have trust in each other. Even the most loving couples find themselves wounded emotionally by conflict; they look to avoid conflict, and to know that when it does occur, they can trust that together they can resolve difficulty equitably (personal communication, Figley, C. R., 2012).

Moral Development in Couple Therapy: A New Approach to Kohlberg's Stages identifies and applies the principles of moral reasoning and development to help couples communicate and resolve differences more effectively. This book is not for counselors and their clients who seek to be guided by a set of rigid rules. Rather, it offers the idea that empathy, guided by mindfulness of the reasoning process itself, gives couples freedom, understanding and flexibility in their decisions. This new approach to couple therapy is a study in fairness, equality, and trust.

Moral development improves trust, trust improves transparency, transparency improves communication, communication improves understanding, understanding improves "innerstanding," empathy and intimacy.

Moral Development in Couple Therapy: A new Approach to Kohlberg's Stages fills a void to provide the rationale for linking the highly respected field of moral development to the field of counseling, specifically in terms of developing trust and intimacy in couples' relationships. Kohlberg's stages of moral judgment and reasoning enable loved ones to determine their individual levels of development and to set meaningful goals. This book also aims to facilitate widespread public education about these matters in order to have the widest impact possible to specifically enhance couples' relationships as well as human interaction worldwide. In that this paradigm is both applicable cross-culturally and to all interpersonal relationships; the couple can be married or not. If married, this book can be useful in developing a more intimate and loving marriage. If not married, the couple might be contemplating marriage or not. If not married but contemplating marriage, this book can be helpful to couples in constructing the foundation for the future of a healthy marriage. If not contemplating, but a couple nevertheless wants to improve their relationship, this information in this book can also set the stage for a healthier relationship. And lastly, since we all interact with others, whether personally or not, this book is for all people to have greater insight into relationships of any kind; it is both applicable cross-culturally and to all interpersonal relationships.

Whether therapeutic, teaching, or empirical research

Go out there and do this!

Notes

1 As the most clearly reflected in thinking, cognition means putting things together, relating events, in cognitive theories, such relating is assumed to be an active connecting process, not a passive connection of events through external association and repetition (Kohlberg, 1972; Galbraith and Jones, 1976).
2 Stages are organized patterns of thinking or reasoning, which represent a hierarchy of increasing cognitive differentiation and integration. Individuals move forward from stage to stage, never backward, and stages cannot be skipped. Lawrence Kohlberg, "Stage and Sequence: The Cognitive-Developmental Approach to Socialization." From the *Handbook of Socialization Theory and Research*, David A. Goslin, p. 376; Galbraith and Jones, 1976.
3 Ibid., p. 338, and p. 352.

Bibliography

Adler, Mortimer J., *Ten Philosophical Mistakes*, New York, Macmillan Publishing Company, 1985.

Archer, Charles A., "'Injustice Anywhere is Injustice Everywhere' In Honor Of Martin Luther King Jr.." *Huff Post*, June 13, 2017.

Aristotle, *Metaphysics*, trans. W.D. Ross, Chicago: William Benton, 1952.

Blasi, A. "Bridging Moral Cognition and Moral Action: A Critical Review of the Literature." *Psychological Bulletin* 88(1980): 1–45.

Branden, Nathaniel, *The Psychology of Self-Esteem*, New York, Bantam Books, 1969.

Brandt, Richard B., *Ethical Theory*, Englewood Cliffs, New Jersey, Prentice- Hall Inc., 1959.

Colby, A., "Evolution of a Moral Developmental Theory." In W. Damon, ed., *New Directions for Child Development: Moral Development*, San Francisco: Josey-Bass, 1978.

Erikson, Erik H., *Childhood and Society*, New York, W.W. Norton and Co., 1968.

Fishkin, James, unpublished doctoral dissertation, Yale University, 1976.

Frankena, W.K., *Ethics*, 1st Ed., Englewood Cliffs, New Jersey, Prentice-Hall, Inc., 1963.

Freud, Sigmund, *The Nature of Illusion*, trans. W.D. Robson-Scott, Garden City, New York, Anchor Books, 1964.

Galbraith, R.E. and Jones, T.E. *Moral Reasoning: A Teaching Handbook for Adapting Kohlberg to the Classroom*, New York: Greenhaven, 1976.

Gibran, Kahlil, *The Prophet*, New York, Alfred A. Knoff, 1965.

Hartshorne, H., and May, M. A., *Studies in the Nature of Character*, Columbia Teacher College. Vol. 1: *Studies in Deceit*. Vol. 2: *Studies in Service and Self-Control*. Vol. 3: *Studies in Organization of Character*, New York: Macmillan, 1928–1930.

King J., Martin Luther, Why We Can't Wait, New York. *The New American Library*, 1963.

Kohlberg, Lawrence, *The Philosophy of Moral Development*, Vol. I, San Francisco, Harper & Row, 1981.

Kohlberg, Lawrence, *Psychology of Moral Development*, Vol. II, San Francisco, Harper & Row, 1984.

Kohlberg, Lawrence, *The Development of Modes of Moral Thinking and Choice in the Years Ten to Sixteen*, unpublished doctoral dissertation," University of Chicago, 1958.

Kohlberg, Lawrence, "Stage and Sequence: The Cognitive Developmental Approach to Socialization." In David Goslin, ed., *Handbook of Socialization Theory and Research*, New York, Rand McNally, 1969.

Kohlberg, Lawrence, *From is to Ought: How to Commit the Naturalistic Fallacy and Get Away with It in the Study of Moral Development, Cognitive Development and Epistemology*, ed. T. Mischel, New York, Academic Press, 1971.

Kohlberg, Lawrence, *"Continuities in Childhood and Adult Moral Development Revisited"*, Life Span Psychology Conference, University of West Virginia, 1972.

Kohlberg, Lawrence, "The Concepts of Developmental Psychology as the Central Guide to Education: Examples from Cognitive, Moral, and Psychological Education." In M.C. Reynolds, ed., *Psychology and the Process of Schooling in the Next Decade: Alternative Conceptions*, Minneapolis, University of Minnesota Press, 1972.

Kohlberg, Lawrence, "The Cognitive Developmental to Moral Education." *The Journal of Philosophy*, October 25, 1973.

Kohlberg, Lawrence, and Gilligan, Carol, "The Adolescent as a Philosopher: The Discovery of Self in a Post-conventional World." *Daedalus*, 100, 1971.

Kohlberg, Lawrence, and Kramer, R., "Richard, Continuities and Discontinuities in Childhood and Adulthood Moral Development, Human Development." *Human Development*, 12(2) 1969.

Lickona, Thomas, *Moral Development and Behavior*, New York, Holt, Rinehart and Winston, 1976.

Nin, Anais, *The Diary of Anais Nin*, ed., Gunther Stuhlmann, Vol. I., New York: The Swallow Press and Harcourt, Brace and World, 1966.

Nin, Anais, *The Diary of Anais Nin*, ed., Gunther Stuhlmann, Vol. II, New York: The Swallow Press and Harcourt, Brace and World, 1967.

Paine, Thomas, *Celestial Tea Box.*

Piaget, J., *The Moral Judgment of the Child*, Glencoe, Illinois: Free Press 1948, 1965, (originally published in 1932).

Plato, *Republic*, trans. Benjamin Jowlett, Chicago, William Benton, 1952.

Plato, *Theaetetus*, Chicago, William Benton, 1852.

Rand, Ayn, *The Ayn Rand Lexicon: Objectivism from A to Z*, New York, New American Library, 1986.

Rawls, John, *Theory of Justice, Cambridge Massachusetts*, Cambridge, MA, The Belknap Press of Harvard University, 1971.

Ries, Steven I., *The Psychological Phenomenon of Moral Relativism and its Relationship to Identity*, Unpublished Qualifying Paper to the Harvard Graduate School of Education, 1979.

Ries, Steven I., *An Empirical Study of an Educational Intervention Curriculum and its Facilitate Effect Upon Moral Development*, doctoral thesis, Harvard, 1981.

Ries, Steven I., "An Intervention Curriculum for Moral Development." *Journal of Moral Education*, 21(1), 1992/2006.

Rest, James, *Development in Judging Moral Issues*, Minnesota, University of Minnesota Press, 1979.

Selman, R.L., *The Growth if Interpersonal Understanding*, New York: Academic Press, 1980.

Shakespeare, William, *The Tragedy of Hamlet, Prince of Denmark*, New Haven, Yale University Press, 1947.

Spinoza, Benedict De, *Ethics*, Chicago, William Benton, 1952.

Trungpa, Chögyam, *Cutting Through Spiritual Materialism*, Berkeley, Shambhala Publications, 1873.

Turiel, Elliot, "Stage Transition in Moral Development." In ed., R.M. Traverse, *Second Handbook of Research on Teaching*, Chicago, Rand McNally and Co., 1972.

Yogananda, Paramahansa, *Autobiography of a Yogi*, Los Angeles, Self-Realization Fellowship, 1979.

Index

Note: Page numbers in **bold** refer to tables.